Help for Your Child

SHARON S. BREHM is Assistant Professor of Psychology at the University of Kansas. She is the author of *The Application of Social Psychology to Clinical Practice* and of a number of papers in scholarly journals.

HELP FOR YOUR CHILD
A Parent's Guide to Mental Health Services

Sharon S. Brehm

A SPECTRUM BOOK

PRENTICE-HALL, INC., *Englewood Cliffs, New Jersey 07632*

Library of Congress Cataloging in Publication Data
BREHM, SHARON S.
  Help for your child.

  (A Spectrum Book)
  Includes index.
  1. Child mental health services.   2. Child psychotherapy.   I. Title.
  RJ111.B72   362.7'8'2   77-28004
  ISBN 0-13-386367-0
  ISBN 0-13-386359-X pbk.

© 1978 by Prentice-Hall, Inc., *Englewood Cliffs, N.J. 07632*

All rights reserved. No part of this book
may be reproduced in any form or
by any means without permission in writing
from the publisher.

A SPECTRUM BOOK

Printed in the United States of America

10 9 8 7 6 5 4 3 2 1

PRENTICE-HALL INTERNATIONAL, INC., *London*
PRENTICE-HALL OF AUSTRALIA PTY. LIMITED, *Sydney*
PRENTICE-HALL, OF CANADA, LTD., *Toronto*
PRENTICE-HALL OF INDIA PRIVATE LIMITED, *New Delhi*
PRENTICE-HALL OF JAPAN, INC., *Tokyo*
PRENTICE-HALL OF SOUTHEAST ASIA PTE. LTD., *Singapore*
WHITEHALL BOOKS LIMITED, *Wellington, New Zealand*

You cannot put a Fire out—
A Thing that can ignite
Can go, itself, without a Fan—
Upon the slowest Night—

You cannot fold a Flood—
And put it in a Drawer—
Because the Winds would find it out—
And tell your Cedar Floor—

Emily Dickinson

Contents

Acknowledgments   *xiii*

1   **INTRODUCTION**   **1**

Who will want to read this book? 5
What information will this book provide? 6
What will a parent know after reading this book? 7

2   **WHEN SHOULD I TAKE MY CHILD TO A MENTAL HEALTH FACILITY?**   **8**

Preschool years, 10
Elementary school years, 20
Adolescence, 26
Collecting information:
    How it can help parents and professionals, 36

3 HOW DO I FIND A MENTAL HEALTH FACILITY? 39

Getting past the emotional barriers, 39
Getting past the practical barriers, 41
A survey of types of mental health facilities, 43

4 WHO WILL I MEET AT A MENTAL HEALTH FACILITY? 50

Major mental health professions, 51
Psychiatrists, 51
Psychologists, 52
Social workers, 53
Mental health workers found primarily
 in inpatient mental health facilities, 54
Allied professions, 55
Concerning the "team" approach, 57

5 HOW WILL A MENTAL HEALTH FACILITY DETERMINE IF MY CHILD NEEDS TREATMENT? 59

Interviews, 59
Intelligence testing, 60
Ability tests, 65
Projective tests, 66
Inventories, 67
Observation, 68
Other types of evaluation processes, 69
Examples of possible evaluations, 70
Mental retardation, 70

6 WHAT KINDS OF TREATMENT MAY A MENTAL HEALTH FACILITY RECOMMEND FOR MY CHILD? 75

No treatment, 76
Modification of parental expectations, 76
Psychotherapy, 78
Behavior therapy, 82

Child-rearing counseling, 85
Supportive therapy, 85
Education, 85
Medication, 87
Inpatient treatment, 88
Supplementary treatments, 90

7 HOW DO I EVALUATE A TREATMENT RECOMMENDED FOR MY CHILD? 92

A note on obtaining "second opinions", 94
Treatment recommendation: No treatment, 96
Treatment recommendation:
  Modification of parental expectations, 96
Treatment recommendation: Psychotherapy, 99
Treatment recommendation: Behavior therapy, 105
Treatment recommendation: Child-rearing counseling, 110
Treatment recommendation: Supportive therapy, 110
Treatment recommendation: Special education, 111
Treatment recommendation: Medication, 113
Treatment recommendation: Inpatient care, 119
Treatment recommendation: Supplementary treatments, 130

8 HOW DO I DISCUSS EVALUATION AND TREATMENT WITH MY CHILD? 132

Explaining why the family is going to a mental health facility, 133
Explaining what will happen at a mental health facility, 135
After the evaluation, 137
Examples of discussing mental health problems with children, 139
The role of other family members, 142

9 HOW DO I PAY FOR MENTAL HEALTH CARE? 144

Outpatient facilities, 144
Inpatient facilities, 148
What does it mean, all this talk about money? 151

10   RIGHTS AND RESPONSIBILITIES   154

Parental rights to professional information—and their responsibilities concerning this information, 155
The rights of children, 157
How to promote quality mental health care for children and families, 161
Urging professionals to provide quality mental health care, 164

Index   167

Acknowledgments

Books somehow always seem inevitable to their authors. You think about something for a long time and then you find yourself writing a book on the subject. The present book is no exception to this general rule. By a series of fortunate circumstances, I encountered three excellent clinical teachers, each of whom stimulated and encouraged my thinking about the role of parents in obtaining mental health services for their children. Their teaching, in combination with my own clinical experiences in a variety of mental health facilities, deeply impressed on me the compelling need for parents to have adequate information. Having learned from and worked with Eric Schopler, Martha Perry, and Beverly VanderVeer LaVeck, this book has seemed inevitable; if I had not met them, I am sure I never would have written it.

In addition to this quality of inevitability, books also share the characteristic of multiplicity of effort, and, again, this book is no exception. Many people from many different walks of life have been generous enough to comment on earlier drafts of the present manuscript. Their comments and suggestions enabled me to progressively improve the accuracy and presentation of the contents of this book. Any remaining inaccuracies or stylistic falls from grace are solely my responsibility and have occurred in spite of the considerable assistance I have had in preparing this book. I am most grateful to the following people for all their help: Glenn Boughton, Melissa Bowerman, John Coie, Lynn Coie, Judith Conger, Gerald Davison, Douglas Denney, Michele Edwards, Raymond Higgins, Beverly VanderVeer LaVeck, Bette Mayhugh, David McAllister, Martha Perry, Robert Schulman, and Nancy Tyler. Special thanks are due to Claudia Citarella of the Spectrum production staff for her hard work on the book and patience with its author.

Help for Your Child

> Dear, dear! How queer everything is today! And yesterday things went on just as usual. I wonder if I've been changed in the night? Let me think: *was* I the same when I got up this morning? I almost think I can remember feeling a little different. But if I'm not the same, the next question is, "Who in the world am I?" Ah, *that's* the great puzzle!
>
> Alice's Adventures in Wonderland,
> Lewis Carroll

Introduction

CHAPTER 1

Parents and children availing themselves of mental health services sometimes feel much like Alice when she fell down the rabbit-hole. As with Alice, there can be confusion at every step of the way. Parents ask themselves, "At what point should I take my child to a mental health facility?" Children ask themselves, "Why are they taking me here?" And these concerns are just the beginning. Once the decision is made to go to a mental health facility, parents must try to find one. Once a facility is located and contact is made, parents and children may meet a variety of mental health professionals, and the variety itself can be quite bewildering. Many people do not know the difference between, for example, psychiatrists and psychologists; moreover, they aren't sure whether they need to know the difference. Long before any of this can be sorted out, vaguely mysterious "evaluation" sessions are scheduled, where important (or so everyone says) "tests" are administered. After this, a conference involving the mental health professional, the parents, and (sometimes) the child will take place and recommendations will be made about what kind of "treatment" the child should receive. If these recommendations are accepted, parents and children

2 Introduction

may soon be involved in any one of a number of types of mental health care, many of which take a long time and are quite expensive.

As can be seen from this very abbreviated sketch of the steps involved in obtaining mental health care for children, obtaining such care is a complicated process. Without sufficient information about what is going on, parents and children may become confused and, not infrequently, fearful. It is difficult for parents and children to know what questions to ask; sometimes they are afraid or embarrassed to ask questions that do come to mind. Many parents hope for "magic" or, at the other extreme, worry that "nothing can be done." Many are too accepting of anything "the doctor says," while many may distrust everything everybody says.

All of this is particularly troublesome in light of the rapid growth of mental health services for children over the last few years. More and more parents and children are now coming into contact with mental health facilities and professionals. Parents may make this contact in an effort to improve the classroom performance of their "learning-disabled" child. Parents may need assistance in coping with their "hyperactive" child. Parents may ask for guidance in changing undesirable behaviors such as bed wetting or excessive aggressiveness. Parents may need evaluations of their child's intellectual functioning because their child's development seems "slow." Parents may have a physically handicapped child who is having emotional difficulties. The list seems almost endless.

In spite of this increased contact, few parents are well informed about the way the mental health system works and what it can do for their children and family. This lack of information, and the confusion and fear it can engender, can have many harmful effects on everyone involved—children, parents, and mental health professionals. Many children probably do not get the mental health care they need because their parents are confused about when mental health services might be helpful and about how to obtain such services. Many parents find it more difficult than it need be to become active, helpful partners in mental health treatment programs for their children. In addition, it is much harder to maintain high standards of professional behavior when the consumers of that behavior are unable to distinguish good care from bad. We have, then, the most unfortunate kind of situation. Parents do not have sufficient information about mental care for children and families, and this lack of information has many undesirable effects. There are several reasons why this state of affairs has come about.

One important reason has to do with the domination of the mental health field by people who have had medical training. The influence of the medical profession has made itself felt in numerous ways. Historically, many of the pioneering writers figures in the field of mental health have been physicians (for example, Sigmund Freud, Carl Jung, and Harry Stack Sullivan). Also, only physicians can administer drugs, and thus, for many people, their primary mental health professional must be a physician. Moreover, while any one mental health facility will have a number of mental health professionals working there (see Chapter 4), the chief administrator is typically a physician. Because of the strong influence of medically trained professionals on the mental health field, mental health care has come to share many of the characteristics of other medical services, and some of these characteristics have hindered providing the public with adequate information about mental health services.

The medical field in general has a long history of authoritarian, "doctor knows best" approaches to "patients." The very use of the word *patient*—a passive recipient of treatment—emphasizes this approach. Informing patients about their treatment has not been greatly emphasized by the medical profession. Doctors are used to saying, "Do this," and their patients are used to saying, "OK." Now, of course, there are reasons why this kind of approach has developed. Doctors are very busy people, and it takes a great deal of time and effort to provide patients with adequate information about their physical condition, the reasons for it, and the treatment that is being recommended. Mental health professionals are also very busy, and it has been only too easy to adopt the medical model of deemphasizing the importance of providing information.

Another reason for the lack of information that the public has received about mental health services involves the lack of a universally agreed-upon understanding among professionals of the nature and causes of mental health problems. There are many different theories about why people become depressed or anxious or aggressive. There are also many different approaches to helping people with such problems. While enormous progress in the understanding of and services for mental health difficulties has occurred in this century, mental health professionals still know distressingly little "for sure" about the psychological functioning of human beings, and some professionals believe they know that one thing is true, while others believe that the exact opposite is true. The mental health field is riddled with controversy and dispute. And it is, of course, rather difficult to give adequate information to the lay public when even the experts disagree among themselves.

Another reason that parents, in particular, have not been well informed about mental health services has to do with the beliefs of some professionals about the role of parents in the development of mental health problems in their children. Some professionals, usually guided by some particular theory about human behavior, have tended to view parental behavior as the cause for the child's developing mental health difficulties. Actually, this is an exceedingly complicated issue. On the one hand, most people—professionals and parents alike—would agree that there are some instances in which bad parenting has led to mental health problems for children. On the other hand, to take this as a *general* proposition without sufficient evidence of its *general* truth is unwarranted and quite unscientific. Fortunately, it appears that mental health professionals are beginning to take a more balanced and objective approach to parents. There is now much more sympathy for parents and much more caution about blaming them for their child's problems. This new professional attitude should be considerably more conducive to providing parents with information.

Finally, it is important that the problem of giving parents information about the mental health system be put in terms of the more general context of having an informed public. In 1951, the psychologist Carl Rogers published a book in which he called his "patients" by the new term *clients*. This change in name had enormous implications that are only beginning to be recognized. A client is one who buys a service; a patient is one who is treated. *Client* denotes an active and, presumably, discriminating consumer who can expect to get his or her money's worth.

It has only been quite recently, however, that anybody was very concerned with helping the consumer make accurate evaluations of what was being purchased. It is not so surprising that parents—the consumers of mental health services for their children—are not very well informed when we realize that it was only within the immediate past that parents, who are also consumers of sleepwear for their children, were informed by manufacturers of the flammable properties of certain sleepwear apparel. It is not surprising that parents are usually totally uninformed about what is entered in their child's record at a mental health facility when we remember that it was only in the early 1970s that consumers were given access to what was entered in their credit-rating records.

Thus, there have been many reasons why the public in general and parents in particular have not been sufficiently informed about mental health care services and procedures. The purpose of this book is to begin to remedy this situation. Addressed specifically to parents, it seeks to provide them with an overall view of what is generally involved in obtaining mental health care for children and families. It has been written in the spirit of consumer advocacy, with the assumption that while a little knowledge may be a dangerous thing, ignorance is certainly dangerous and adequate knowledge can only be beneficial.

WHO WILL WANT TO READ THIS BOOK?

Mental health care for children differs in many respects from that for adults. One very important difference is that, most typically, the child does not decide to go to a mental health facility; moreover, frequently the child has little to say about whether the recommendations received are carried out. A family may go to a mental health facility because of the *child's* problems, but it is the *parents* who make most of the crucial decisions about where and when to go, and about how they will respond to the advice they receive at the facility.

Thus, this book is written primarily for parents who are thinking about taking their child to a mental health facility, who are going to one already, or who have been to one in the past. Every child and every family is different, with different problems and with different resources available to them. This book attempts a general overview that should be of some interest to every reader, but individual parents probably will find some specific aspects more useful than others. It is recommended that parents who are interested, for whatever reason, in mental health facilities for children first read the entire book to gain an overall perspective. After this, they may want to reread specific sections that are of particular interest to them.

This book is designed to be as useful as possible to the parent who may need to have contact with the mental health system. One procedure that is strongly recommended throughout the book is that parents question any mental health professional with whom they are working about anything and everything that confuses them, puzzles them, or simply interests them. To make this process easier, examples of possible questions that parents may want to ask are provided in various chapters.

If the mental health system is frequently confusing to parents, it can be even more often confusing and frightening to children. Parents who take their child to a mental health facility need to be able to discuss what's going on both with the child and with any brothers or sisters in the family. A specific chapter has been provided to help parents discuss mental health issues with their children.

Furthermore, some parents may want to discuss specific details presented in this book with their children. This is left to the individual parent's discretion, but such discussions would seem especially useful with older children. Indeed, for older adolescents who read reasonably well, parents may want to suggest that they too read this book. Then parents and child can discuss their reactions to the book together. This kind of approach should help avoid many problems of communication that might otherwise occur, and can lay the foundation for the sort of cooperative effort that will be of vast benefit to the entire family.

In addition to parents and children, some professionals may want to be familiar with the contents of this book. It may help remind them of issues and concerns that can arise and that they will want to discuss with their clients. Again, a joint reading project may be beneficial, this time with clients and professionals reading the book and then discussing it together. This discussion could be utilized as an opportunity for a professional to outline specific aspects of his or her approach that may differ from the general characteristics described in this book.

WHAT INFORMATION WILL THIS BOOK PROVIDE?

This book is organized as a consumer's guide to mental health facilities. It will take the reader step by step through the typical procedures that occur at most such facilities. We will begin at the beginning—with considering when parents might wish to take their child to a mental health facility. Then we will discuss how parents can find a mental health facility that is appropriate for their family, what kinds of professionals work at mental health facilities, how mental health professionals determine if the child and/or family needs treatment, what kinds of treatment programs may be recommended, and how parents can evaluate the treatment that is offered. In addition, there are chapters describing the ways in which mental health care can be paid for and the rights and responsibilities parents have in providing good mental health care for children.

Since this book is meant primarily for the lay public, it has been written as much as possible in everyday, nonprofessional language. Where the use of professional terminology has been unavoidable, such terms are defined in the text. References to professional publications have been kept at a minimum, but are cited when it is necessary to draw the reader's attention to scientific findings.

WHAT WILL A PARENT KNOW AFTER READING THIS BOOK?

To be a parent of a child who has mental health problems *is* to bear a kind of resemblance to Alice in Wonderland. Things do seem different and strange and, sometimes, frightening. This book cannot make these feelings disappear. It can remind parents that they are still parents, that their child is still their child, and that even Wonderlands are easier to get through if you have a map.

Using this book as a map—finding out the "lay of the land" of the mental health system—should enable parents to ask sensible questions of professionals and to discuss important issues intelligently with them. This does not mean that reading this book will make a parent into a professional; it will not. Experts will still be experts, and their expertise is a most valuable commodity. This book seeks to assist parents in making the best possible use of this expertise. Only when parents are equipped with sufficient information can they make sure they receive the best possible professional help. When parents are informed, rather than bewildered, they can be active, helpful participants in providing mental health care for their child.

> "Seven years and six months!" Humpty Dumpty repeated thoughtfully. "An uncomfortable sort of age. Now if you'd asked *my* advice, I'd have said 'Leave off at seven'—but it's too late now."
> "I never ask advice about growing," Alice said indignantly.
> "Too proud?" the other enquired.
>
> *Through the Looking-Glass*

When Should I Take My Child to a Mental Health Facility?

CHAPTER 2

The first step parents must take in obtaining mental health care for their child is actually making the decision that their child needs such care. As it turns out, this is no easy decision. Childhood is a time of growth and change. All children have some difficulties at some times. How is a parent to decide when a problem is more than just a part of the normal ups and downs of childhood and adolescence?

While there is no simple answer to this question, some general principles can help. First, parents should trust their own feelings. Probably the best guide to when something is really wrong is when the parent *feels* that something is wrong. Parents usually have good common sense about their children and they should rely on this common sense. For instance, virtually all parents react to a problem in terms of its *duration*. If fifteen-year-old Kathy appears depressed and withdrawn for a few days, most parents would be concerned and try their best to be helpful; few parents would, however, see this as sufficient reason to decide to take Kathy to see a mental health professional. Only when the problem continues past what the parent considers to be the normal or typical time period for Kathy

8

have these feelings will consulting a mental health facility become something to consider seriously.

Or take the *intensity* of a behavior. If eight-year-old Johnny strikes out in an angry, but really rather halfhearted fashion, against a playmate, most parents would express concern, but, again, few would think they should go to a mental health clinic for assistance. On the other hand, if the same child became absolutely enraged and acted in a way that could (or does) seriously injure the other child, then most parents would become very worried and would think about talking with a mental health professional. In this instance, the duration or frequency of the behavior is not important; what is important is that the intensity of the behavior exceeds the parent's common sense notion of what is reasonable behavior under the circumstances.

Another factor that parents will take into consideration in evaluating the seriousness of a suspected problem is the *age* of the child. Few parents would worry about a ten-month-old child who does not use words; many parents would be very concerned about a thirty-month-old child who does not use words. While there are no rigid rules for exactly when a child should speak — or do anything else — there are some general expectations as to the timing of many aspects of development.

It should be realized that there is no real substitute for this commonsense parental knowledge. There certainly is not now, and probably never will be, any way for mental health professionals to set up clear, explicit, and absolute guidelines as to when a specific parent should take a specific child to a mental health facility. The first, most basic, and irreplaceable ingredient in making a wise decision about this is the parent's common sense knowledge about children in general and the specific child in particular.

In addition to this basic knowledge, however, parents can seek out more detailed information. For example, you can be much more effective and accurate in evaluating the seriousness of your child's problem if you have a good understanding of normal development. One of the best ways to achieve this understanding is to have raised several children; indeed, parents who have had a number of children tend to be pretty sophisticated about knowing when there is or is not cause for serious concern. Unfortunately, parents with their first child do not have the benefit of this experience. Furthermore, it has been my personal observation that some parents simply find it easy to understand their child (and children in general), while others find this a more difficult undertaking. I don't know why this is, but I do believe that this difference exists. At any rate, parents who believe that, for whatever reason, they need to increase their knowledge about children have a number of ways to get more information. They can talk with parents who have a number of children; they can read books or take courses on child development; they can talk with an expert on children such as a pediatrician, or a mental health professional, or a teacher who specializes in the field of child development.

Another type of information that can be helpful to parents in evaluating possible problems involves finding out about the types of mental health problems that children have. This information will, of course, be general and usually cannot serve to describe precisely any individual child. Sensibly used, however, information about children's mental health problems can alert parents to general areas of possible difficulty. There are many possible sources of information about the mental health problems of children: courses are offered in most colleges and universities; parent effectiveness training (PET) courses offered at many community mental health clinics usually provide some discussion of children's mental health problems; experts are available for consultation; books can be found in any library.

This chapter provides a brief summary of the most typical kinds of children's mental health problems. For additional information, parents should consult any of the sources noted in the previous discussion. In particular, I would recommend two books that offer excellent coverage of their topics: (1) *Child Behavior* by F. Ilg and L. Ames (New York: Harper & Row, 1955) for an overview of normal child development, and (2) *Child Psychopathology* by M. Erickson (Englewood Cliffs, N.J.: Prentice-Hall, 1977) for a more detailed discussion of children's mental health problems.

For assistance in reading the following summary of children's mental health problems, Table 2-1 should be consulted. This table indicates that the summary is organized by age group, with the three main divisions being the preschool years, elementary school age, and adolescence. Within each age division, a number of mental health problems are described; a checkmark in the table indicates that the particular problem is described for that particular age group. I recommend that the reader first read the entire summary straight through in order to get a general overview; parts of more specific interest can then be reread with the benefit of the context obtained from the first reading.

PRESCHOOL YEARS

The preschool years are a time of rapid growth and frequent change. There are always many "problems" during these years, from feeding to

TABLE 2-1
Mental Health Problems of Children Discussed in This Book

	Preschool Years	Elementary School Age	Adolescence
Intellectual Development/ Mental Retardation	✓	✓	✓
Learning Disabilities		✓	✓
Psychosis		✓	
Autism	✓		
Childhood schizophrenia	✓		
Schizophrenia			✓
Manic-depression			✓
Emotional Disturbances	✓	✓	✓
School phobia		✓	
Behavior Problems			
Eating	✓	✓	✓
Toilet-training or elimination	✓	✓	
Sleep	✓	✓	✓
Aggression	✓	✓	✓
Timidity	✓	✓	✓
Hyperactivity	✓	✓	
Sexual difficulties			✓
Drug-related problems			✓
Communication Disorders		✓	
Articulation	✓		
Stuttering	✓		✓
Speech delay	✓		
Developmental aphasia	✓		
Traumatic brain injury			✓
Problems of Physically Handicapped Children	✓	✓	✓

toilet-training to learning to cross the street. In most cases, such problems can be handled by parents, perhaps with advice from family, friends, pediatricians, and so on. Other problems, however, may require the assistance of mental health professionals.

Intellectual Development

Not all children develop intellectually at the same rate. Some children develop quickly and, for example, may start speaking quite early. Others develop more slowly. In addition, of course, some children are more intelligent than others, and children differ in the ways that they are intelligent. These are all variations that are quite normal.

Sometimes, however, parents become concerned that their child is not developing normally in intellectual functioning. There are two times when this concern is most likely to occur. The first period is at birth or shortly thereafter. Some children are born with physical disorders that are usually associated with some degree of mental retardation. These types of disorders include the following

- *Down's syndrome:* a genetic abnormality (usually *not* inherited), frequently called mongolism.
- *Hydrocephaly (primary type:)* enlargement of skull due to fluid accumulation within the brain.
- *PKU (phenylketonuria:)* a metabolic disorder that may now be treated by a diet; when promptly initiated after birth, this diet greatly reduces the pos- that a child with PKU will be mentally retarded.

These types of physical disorders are relatively easy to detect. Children with Down's syndrome or hydrocephaly have distinct physical characteristics that the obstetrician and pediatrician will recognize. PKU is detected through a simple test routinely carried out by hospitals.[1] While the mental retardation that can result from such physical disorders can be extremely difficult for parent and child to cope with, its relatively easy identification makes parents' decisions about seeking assistance from mental health professionals more or less automatic. Such a child will, as a matter of course, be under a physician's care, and most physicians will recommend the assistance of mental health professionals in evaluating the child's intellectual development and planning for the child's education and care. If, for any reason, this recommendation is not given, parents should ask the physician about it; if necessary, they should consult a mental health professional without a recommendation from the physician.

Another time when many parents become concerned about their preschooler's intellectual development is when the child is around eighteen to twenty-four months old and the parent expects the child to begin talking.

[1]However, parents should be aware that this screening procedure does result in some "false positives"—that is, children who have a temporary condition (transiently elevated plasma phenylalanine concentrations) which is *mis*diagnosed as PKU. For such false positives, the special diet is harmful rather than helpful. To avoid misdiagnosis, parents should insist on careful follow-up evaluations if routine screening indicates their child has PKU.

If the child does not, the parent may begin to worry. This worry needs to be evaluated in light of the family context. If there are other children, did they also speak late? Did the parents or their brothers or sisters begin to speak somewhat later than usual? If there is a history in the family of late development of speech, the child may just be following the family pattern and may catch up to normal levels fairly soon. Parents also need to consider the overall pattern of the child's development. Did the child walk late, too? Does the child seem to have trouble understanding gestures as well as speech? Is the child sluggish and apathetic? Does he or she drool excessively? If there seems to be a general pattern of slow development, parents should consult their pediatrician. If the pediatrician believes that the child is having difficulties in intellectual development, he or she will usually recommend that the parent consult a mental health professional to have the child's intellectual development evaluated. If the pediatrician does not recommend this, but the parents continue to be concerned about the child's intellectual growth, they should consult a mental health professional on their own initiative.

Psychosis

Psychosis indicates an extreme disturbance in accurately perceiving reality and in responding emotionally to this reality. It is a very severe mental health problem. Fortunately, childhood psychosis is rare and should be fairly easy to recognize. Unfortunately, some parents may try to convince themselves that everything will be all right and delay getting assistance for their child—psychotic children need help and they need it as soon as possible. Although different terms have been used to describe psychotic children (including *atypical child, symbiotic psychosis,* and *childhood psychosis*), the two most common labels are *autism* and *childhood schizophrenia.*

AUTISM

Children who are considered to be autistic typically display at least some of the following behavior patterns. It is said that, as babies, autistic children do not make themselves ready to be picked up. They may fight being picked up or they may just lay passively, but they do not show the usual adjustment behavior (holding up their arms, molding their bodies to whomever picks them up) shown by normal infants. Unfortunately, most of the evidence about this behavior is collected after the child is much older and the mother is looking back on the infancy period. It is uknown how many perfectly normal children may display the same type of behavior. If, however, the baby's not becoming ready to be picked up is persistant and worries the parent, it is worth a trip to the pediatrician to inquire about it.

More worrisome to many parents, and probably more likely to indicate that something really is wrong, is the autistic infant's lack of response to the human environment. The autistic infant may be fascinated by small things (changes of light, scratching on the crib), but not respond to people (or, in some instances, to animals). If this lack of response continues, parents frequently are concerned that the child is deaf or mentally retarded. This concern should, of course, be promptly checked out.

It is usually during the ages from two to five that autistic behavior becomes most evident. Autistic children appear extremely aloof from other people. They may be fascinated by mechanical objects, such as record players, but will typically not even make eye contact with other people. Some autistic children show severe resistance to any kind of change. The slightest rearrangement of their toys, for example, will occasion a violent temper tantrum. Food preferences also tend to be terribly strong and accompanied by temper tantrums whenever any food other than the preferred item is urged upon them.

Autistic children always have extreme difficulties with speech. Some autistic children remain mute for life. Others talk gibberish (it sounds something like speech, but is not), or repeat things other people say, or *always* call themselves "you" rather than "I." These speech difficulties do not necessarily mean that a child is autistic, but if they persist, the parent should consider having the child evaluated at a mental health facility or speech clinic.

In summary, the typical autistic child will not relate to other people, will throw violent temper tantrums when things are changed, and will have severe speech problems. Any one of these behaviors should concern a parent. All of these behaviors combined suggest that something is seriously wrong and should occasion immediate attention by both parents and professionals.

CHILDHOOD SCHIZOPHRENIA

This group of children is somewhat more difficult to describe. The behaviors that characterize these children are not as well agreed upon as those that characterize autistic children. Schizophrenic children are perhaps best characterized as "strange." They seem to be aware of other people, but they react strangely to them: they may ignore them, touch them inappropriately, or cling to them. They may talk, but use language primarily to communicate fantasies or delusions. They may engage in self-destructive behavior. They may become preoccupied with special objects or with certain daily routines. They may develop excessive fears. In general appearance, the schizophrenic child is withdrawn from and disinterested in the "real world" and preoccupied with an "inner world" of fears and fantasies.

These behaviors are usually not recognizable during infancy (indeed, some believe that childhood schizophrenia does not exist in infants). But, by ages three to five, the behaviors become apparent. The parent whose child shows strange behaviors and extreme withdrawal from the real world should see a mental health professional without delay. The child may or may not be schizophrenic, but it is highly likely that there is a serious problem of some sort.

Emotional Disturbances

Even very young children have their fair share of emotional upsets. Children can become very sad when a family member or cherished pet dies; they can become fearful about specific objects that do not frighten other children; they can become angry or frustrated and scream and throw themselves on the floor. Fortunately, these disturbances usually are of relatively short duration and parents are able to help the child get through such distrubances without seeking professional assistance. Sometimes, however, help is needed. Some children mourn the death of a loved one for such a long time that parents become concerned. Some children do not outgrow their fears. Some children have many, many temper tantrums of great intensity. Moreover, some children seem emotionally upset, but their parents cannot figure out anything that might have caused this. Whenever parents feel that their child has been emotionally upset for too long a time (for this individual child, for his or her age group), they should seriously consider consulting a mental health professional.

Behavior Problems

Every child has behavior problems at one time or another. Some eat poorly; others sleep badly; some have difficulty with toilet-training; some children are too aggressive, while others are too timid, and others are too active. Most behavior problems occur for a while and then fade away as the child grows up and parents and child learn to modify their behavior in accordance with each other. Some behavior problems, however, do not go away by themselves. It is these that should lead a parent to consider taking the child to a mental health facility.

EATING

The child who has eating problems should first be brought to a pediatrician, who knows what a child should eat and what weight is appropriate. If the pediatrician's suggestions fail to solve the problem, the pediatrician and the parents should consider consulting a mental health professional. For some eating problems, perhaps especially overeating, early work with a mental health professional may prevent later, more severe problems.

TOILET-TRAINING

Problems with toilet-training should first be discussed with a pediatrician. It is important that a thorough physical examination be conducted. The pediatrician can also help the parent know what to expect in terms of typical problems with toilet-training. If the physical examination reveals no organic problem and toilet-training problems persist beyond what the parent considers reasonable, the parent will want to think about consulting a mental health professional.

SLEEP DISTURBANCES

Again, the pediatrician should be the first expert consulted. Also, it is very important to talk with the child about why he or she is having trouble sleeping. Some sleep problems can be solved by simple remedies such as leaving on a night light for a child who is troubled by the dark. If the child is physically normal and simple remedies do not work, the parent will want to think about going to a mental health facility.

AGGRESSION

Parents usually attempt to handle excessive aggression on their own, without expert help, and usually they succeed. Sometimes, however, problems with aggression continue in spite of the parents' best efforts to control the child. Aggression is one of those behaviors that may be much easier to change early in the child's development and much more difficult to change later on. The parent who is concerned about a child's level of aggressive behavior should not hesitate to discuss it with a mental health professional.

TIMIDITY

Some children are very timid. They may avoid others (both adults and peers), may cling to their parents, and may have many fears. As with aggression, parents may be able to work out ways to decrease the child's timidity by themselves. If not, consultation with mental health professionals should be considered.

HYPERACTIVITY

Hyperactivity is just what the name implies: an excess of activity. This problem has received much attention in the last few years, and there are now quite a few children who have been labeled "hyperactive." In spite of (or perhaps because of) this new-found popularity, hyperactivity is a controversial subject. Behavior that some parents and professionals consider hyperactive may not be so considered by other parents and professionals. This controversy is especially important in that a typical treatment for hyperactivity is medication, and any medication may have some undesirable side effects. (We will discuss issues concerning treatment of hyperactivity later in this book.)

The acutely hyperactive child is characterized by an inability to remain still for any substantial period of time, by the tendency to become easily distracted, and by difficulty in persisting in a given activity. Usually, these problems are more in evidence during the school years than at younger ages, but they certainly can be displayed during the preschool period. If a parent notices that (1) the child is extremely restless and can't seem to pay attention to any one thing, (2) these problems persist over a long time, and (3) the problems occur without any clear relationship to outside influences (it's perfectly normal for a child to show these behaviors at some times—for example, when anticipating an exciting trip away from home), then the parent may well want to have the child evaluated.

Again, the first expert to be consulted is the pediatrician. Because of the controversy surrounding the identification and treatment of hyperactivity, however, parents should feel free to consult more than one person. For example, if the pediatrician thinks the child is not hyperactive, but the parent is still concerned, than a mental health professional should be consulted. If, on the other hand, the pediatrician believes the child to be hyperactive, the parent may well wish to consult a mental health professional for a second opinion, especially before agreeing to place the child on medication.

Communication Disorders

One of the more common problem areas of early childhood involves communication difficulties. Mentally retarded children as well as psychotic children frequently have communication problems. In addition, there are many children who are not mentally retarded or psychotic, but who do have difficulties in speaking and/or in the use of language. It should be noted that any parent who becomes concerned about a child's communication skills should first make sure the child receives a thorough physical examination, including a hearing test. Sometimes apparent speech or language problems are related to some physical problem, such as difficulty in hearing.

ARTICULATION

Some children have difficulty pronouncing words properly. Such difficulties are, of course, quite typical when the child is first beginning to speak. If articulation problems persist and are bothersome to the child, the parent may wish to take the child to a speech clinic for an evaluation.

STUTTERING

Stuttering can be a normal part of the development of speech. Most young children who stutter will not continue to stutter when they are older. In fact, parents should be careful *not* to make the very young child self-conscious by drawing attention to his or her stuttering. If a young child who is still developing language skills begins to stutter, the best approach to take is simply to ignore the stuttering. When stuttering continues for a long time and/or is extremely severe, however, the parent may wish to take the child to a speech clinic for an evaluation.

Speech problems are considered to be relevant to the mental health of the child primarily because of the emotional problems that can be associated with difficulties in speaking. Although these emotional effects tend to be greater with older children, even young children who speak especially oddly or poorly can become embarrassed, begin to avoid speaking, and, sometimes, begin to avoid other people, especially peers who may make fun of them. Speech and langauge specialists will be able to assist the child with any specific speech problem and they tend to be sensitive to and helpful with the emotional effects of the speech problem. If, however, emotional problems persist and are of concern to the parent, consultation with a mental health professional is recommended.

SPEECH DELAY

The rate of development of speech varies tremendously from child to child. Some children are "fast talkers," while others are "slow talkers." This kind of variation is perfectly normal. Sometimes, however, there are children with more severe speech delays. These children appear to learn to talk *much* more slowly than would be expected for their age. If a parent becomes concerned about a child's slowness in developing speech, consultation with a speech clinic should be considered. The speech clinic can determine whether or not the child's speech is seriously delayed. If there is a delay, a variety of factors may be involved (for example, mental retardation, too much pressure being placed on the child to speak, specific language disability of unknown origin), and mental health professionals frequently become involved in trying to determine the exact nature of the problem.

DEVELOPMENTAL APHASIA

When a child has severe difficulties in the use of language and is not mentally retarded, sensorily impaired (for example, hard of hearing), or emotionally disturbed (for example, autistic), then some professionals would term the child's problem *developmental aphasia*. This term indicates that some kind of impairment to the child's central nervous system is postulated, although only some of the children so diagnosed show actual evidence of such an impairment. Because of the inferential nature of the term, some professionals prefer not to use the label *developmental asphasia* and, instead, use the term *verbal communication disorder*. Regardless of the confusion about the exact nature of this disorder and what it should be called, there is considerable agreement that some children do have severe language difficulties who are not mentally retarded, sensorily impaired, or emotionally disturbed.

There is also considerable agreement about the kinds of language difficulties that are usually involved. Severe language disorders are characterized by at least some of the following behaviors: speech delay, inconsistent responses to sound (for example, turning in the direction of a soft noise but not a loud one), unusual use of words (for example, calling a kettle "to make a cup of tea," calling a hospital "horse-a-petal"), confusion of different meanings of a word, reduction of words and sentences to syllables or words, and echolalia (repetition of what has been said by oneself or by others). While all of these behaviors can be found in normal young children as they develop their use of language, speech disordered children are identifiable by the persistence of extreme language difficulties. Children who display such persistant and extreme problems in speaking should be evaluated at a speech clinic. For those children who do have a severe language impairment, life can be extremely frustrating and confusing. Parents of such a child may wish to obtain advice from mental health professionals on how to assist their child's emotional and social development.

Physically Handicapped Children

Children with physical handicaps have unique problems to face in growing up. They have, on the one hand, the problem of coping with their disability. Parents are usually well alerted to such specific problems and avail themselves of the needed medical and educational assistance. In addition to coping with the disability itself, emotional and/or behavioral problems may arise. If this occurs, the parent should strongly consider obtaining professional assistance in coping with them. Most medical and educational personnel who work with handicapped children are aware of the possibility of emotional or behavioral problems and will themselves be able to help the parents or refer the parents to someone else for assistance.

ELEMENTARY SCHOOL YEARS

Mental Retardation

While most of the more severe forms of mental retardation are recognized before the child goes to school, some of the milder forms may not be recognized until school age. Typically, children are given some type of intelligence test in school and, just as typically, these tests are administered to children in groups rather than individually. If as the result of such a test or as the result of the observations by themselves or by the child's teacher, parents become concerned about their child's intellectual functioning, they should talk with the child's teacher or the school psychologist if one is available. An important general principle is that neither the results of group testing nor the child's performance in the classroom should be used as the sole basis for identifying mental retardation. The child must be given an individually administered intelligence test and the results of this test carefully considered in light of the child's behavior at home and in school. This type of evaluation requires a psychologist.[2] If a school psychologist is available, the parents may be able to have this person conduct the individual testing and overall evaluation. If, however, *for any reason* the parents cannot or do not want to have this done by a school psychologist (for example, if there is no school psychologist; or if there is one, but this person prefers to have others administer individual tests; or if there is one, but the parents and/or the child do not feel sufficiently comfortable with this person) then parents can consult a psychologist outside the school setting. This psychologist can then assist the parents and child in discussing with school personnel the child's intellectual functioning and the type of educational program that will be needed to maximize the child's growth.

Learning Disabilities

Perhaps the most typical mental health problem that arises in the elementary school age years is that of learning disability. While there is much controversy over how learning disabilities come about, most people are able to agree on what constitutes a learning disability. The usual definition is that a learning-disabled child is a child with normal sight and hearing who scores in the normal (or superior) range on an intelligence test, but who performs below normal in the classroom.

For this definition to apply, the child's sight and hearing must first be determined to be in the normal range. For the second part of this definition — the child's score on an intelligence test — all that was stated above in regard to intelligence testing applies here. An intelligence test must be individually administered to the child by a psychologist.

The third aspect of the definition is more complex. Children can fail to perform at the level of their abilities for many reasons. They can be unhappy at school, they can be unhappy at home, they can have an inadequate teacher, they can have some specific problem in learning, or they can have some combination of these problems. Obviously, then, in order to help such children someone will have to sort through all these various possibilities and devise a program, either for the home, the school, or both, to assist these children to perform at an academic level more consistent with their

---

[2]The training and skills of psychologists as well as other mental health professionals are described in Chapter 4.

abilities. This someone will also have to coordinate what goes on at home with what goes on at school.

Some school systems have school psychologists who are quite expert at working with learning-disabled children and can provide this kind of complex assistance: evaluating the problem, devising a treatment program, and coordinating its implementation. In some school systems, however, this kind of person is not available and parents will need to go to a mental health facility for this assistance.

Psychosis

While many children who have psychotic problems are identified prior to attending school, some develop psychotic behavior—or at least it is recognized as such—during the elementary school years. Usually, such problems would be of the schizophrenic type, and the symptoms would be similar to those described for the preschool years. Parents who are concerned because their child shows some of the strange and extreme behaviors that can be associated with childhood schizophrenia should immediately have their child evaluated by a mental health professional.

Emotional Disturbances

When children are worried or fearful or angry, they can express their feelings in many ways. Sometimes their sleep is disturbed; sometimes their school performance suffers; sometimes their usual eating habits are disrupted. When the emotional state of the child is reflected in his or her behavior in such ways, parents will frequently first notice the specific problem behavior, since the feelings of the child may be more difficult to detect. Descriptions of such problems are given in the following section on behavior problems. Sometimes, however, parents become aware of the child's feelings without having concerns about a specific behavior. They may notice that their child has become quite tense and preoccupied or that the child seems highly fearful (either in general or about objects that do not make other children fearful) or that their child seems sad and unhappy. As we noted in the discussion of preschoolers' emotional problems, many such emotional disturbances are transitory, and parents will be able to help their child get through them without obtaining professional assistance. When, however, an emotional difficulty endures beyond what the parents feel is a reasonable time, then consultation with a mental health professional is recommended.

SCHOOL PHOBIA

One of the most common emotional disturbances in childhood is school phobia. The identifying characteristic of this problem is quite obvious: the child stops going to school. Frequently, the child seems highly fearful when the parents urge that he or she go back to school; in addition, physical illness is often involved. Some children pretend to be ill as an excuse to stay out of school; others display physical symptoms (for example, vomiting, diarrhea) indicating that they are experiencing great stress. Whatever the exact pattern of the child's behavior, parents should become concerned whenever their child seems upset by the prospect of going to school and stops attending school.

When a child stops going to school, parents should immediately try to find out from the child why he or she wants to stay home. Sometimes there are realistic reasons for the child's behavior (such as a teacher who upsets the child or a classmate who bullies him or her) that parents can have corrected. Sometimes, however, the child cannot explain his or her behavior, and the parents are unable to figure out what's causing it. In the absence of any identifiable cause for the child's behavior, parents can simply urge the child to return to school; with some children, this will be more effective if the parents also promise to grant the child some desirable activity or object upon the child's return to school. Unfortunately, urging and promising rewards will not always suffice to get the child back into school. At this point, parents should immediately consult a mental health professional. School phobia is a fairly common psychological problem with children during the elementary school years, and it usually responds quickly to professional treatment. The danger of school phobia is that the longer the child is out of school, the more difficult it becomes to get the child to go back. Parents should always deal with school avoidance. Frequently their own efforts will be successful, but if these initial efforts do not succeed, immediate professional intervention is necessary.

Behavior Problems

Behavior problems are at least as prevalent in the elementary school age years as in the early years. Their focus, however, tends to change. In general, there is less concern with the basic functions of eating, sleeping, and elimination and more concern with the child's social interactions and learning experiences.

EATING

Eating can be a problem for elementary-school-age children. Some become obese; some become quite thin; some become terribly finicky and will eat only a few foods. If an eating problem continues over a fairly lengthy period of time and the parent has concerns about the child's nutrition and health, the parent should check first with the child's pediatrician. If there are no physical problems, but the eating behavior continues to cause trouble for the child and/or family, the parent may wish to consult a mental health professional.

ELIMINATION

It is not that rare for young elementary-school-age boys (around ages six to eight) to have some difficulty with bed wetting. This is less common for girls and it is more unusual for both boys and girls to have problems with soiling. If a child has a mild problem with enuresis (involuntary urination), the parent should discuss this with the child's pediatrician; often some common sense advice that the pediatrician has found useful with other children will be sufficient to solve the problem. If the child's enuresis is more severe or if soiling is involved, the parent will want to have the child undergo a physical exam, and then, if this exam does not reveal any physical problem and the elimination difficulty persists, consult a mental health professional.

SLEEPING

It is perfectly normal for children of this age group to have nightmares or, from time to time, difficulty sleeping. If, however, any sleeping problem persists or is quite severe, the parent will want to consider seeing the pediatrician and then, if the problem persists, a mental health professional.

AGGRESSION

Excessive aggression is one of the most frequently seen behavior problems in children of the elementary-school-age years, especially in males. If parents feel their child is too aggressive with peers, with siblings (brothers or sisters), or even with animals, or if a teacher reports the child as being overly aggressive at school, the parents well want to see a mental health professional. Often it is fairly easy to help the child reduce this aggression, and it is usually the case that the younger the child, the easier this is. Also, of course, it is always possible that the child's aggression is perfectly normal, but that parents or teachers have unrealistic expectations. In these circumstances, an outside expert is needed to help the people involved gain some perspective on what amount of aggression can be expected, and to help them tolerate normal levels of aggression.

TIMIDITY

In our society at present there are sex differences in certain problems that children tend to have. Boys tend to have problems with aggression and girls with timidity. Regardless of the sex of the child and regardless of the specific behavior—aggression or withdrawal—the same comments apply. A mental health professional can be of assistance in helping an overly aggressive or timid child, and in setting realistic expectations for adults about what levels of aggression or timidity should be acceptable.

HYPERACTIVITY

Hyperactivity is another behavior problem that is frequently found in elementary-school-age children. The same principles that applied to characterizing a preschooler as hyperactive also apply here. Deciding whether a child is hyperactive is best done in consultation with a mental health professional. The opinions of parents, teachers, or pediatricians are important but need to be augmented with an evaluation by a mental health professional.

Frequently, the child who is considered hyperactive also will be viewed as having a learning disability. This connection is a rather obvious one, since any child who is restless, easily distracted, and does not persist in a given task will have great difficulty learning adequately. However, not every child who has a learning problem necessarily displays excessive activity. A very quiet, placid child can still have problems in learning. Both possible difficulties—excessive activity and learning problems—should be considered separately and need to be evaluated by a mental health professional.

Communication Disorders

Communication problems found in elementary-school-age children are not significantly different from those found in preschool children. The discussion of these problems as they might occur in preschool children can also be utilized for consideration of elementary-school-age children.

Physically Handicapped Children

Physically handicapped children of elementary school age have a variety of difficulties to surmount: they need an educational setting that will maximize their learning; they need social interaction with their peers; and they still have the special problems in living that their specific disability brings about. Having to surmount all these difficulties simultaneously often is very stressful for the child and the family, and can create emotional and/or behavioral problems. As noted earlier, if emotional or behavioral problems do arise, the parent should consider obtaining assistance in coping with them. This assistance may be available from the medical and educational personnel who are already working with the child, or it may be necessary to consult a mental health professional for additional assistance.

ADOLESCENCE

Mental Retardation

During the adolescent years, the major concerns for parents of mentally retarded children are to cope with behavior problems that can arise during these years and to prepare the child and themselves for the child's future. Not uncommonly, one of the most difficult areas to deal with during these years is the child's sexual development. In dealing with sexual behavior, or any other behavior that is of concern to the parent and/or the child, parents should feel free to consult a mental health professional. Mentally retarded children are similar to handicapped children: they may have problems that arise, at least in part, from the special difficulties their handicap brings. If parents can cope with such problems by themselves, this is admirable, but it is equally admirable for a parent to seek expert assistance to help make the child's and the family's life as pleasant and rewarding as possible.

The other major concern that parents have to face with adolescents who are mentally retarded is making plans for their future. Often this can be done in consultation with other agencies or professionals (for example, parents' groups, lawyers, employment agencies such as Goodwill Industries), but sometimes the factual and emotional turmoil involved in making and carrying out such plans creates severe stress for the parents. At such times, parents should not hesitate to consult mental health professionals who are expert in the field of mental retardation. These professionals will be able to provide the parent with information and will assist the parent in working through both factual and emotional confusion.

Learning Disabilities

One always hopes that learning problems will be identified in the early elementary school years. If they are not recognized then, but persist without remedial attention into the adolescent years, the child is likely to have had years of frustration and failure. These years may lead some children to think badly of themselves (have "low self-esteem") and/or to think badly of school. A large number of "high school dropouts" may in fact be children who have had learning difficulties that were never treated and that led them to hate the school situation and to get away from it at the earliest opportunity.

If parents of an adolescent become concerned that their teenager is showing learning difficulties *above and beyond some temporary rebellion and loss of interest in schooling,* then the parents should talk with the child's principal and teachers. If the school personnel also feel that the child may have learning difficulties (or even if they do not believe this, but the parents observe that the child's difficulties persist), then the parents should contact a mental health facility. It can often come as a distinct relief to a child to learn that his or her difficulties are not because of being "dumb," but because of specific learning problems that usually can be helped by participating in special learning programs.

Psychosis

The types of psychoses that were described earlier occur during the preadolescent years. During the adolescent period, the features of severe emotional disturbance are quite different and begin to resemble the features of severe emotional disturbance found in adults. There are two main types that should be considered: schizophrenia and manic-depression.

SCHIZOPHRENIA
Adolescents who are undergoing a schizophrenic episode may show a variety of unusual behaviors. They may become excessively withdrawn,

not interacting with other people and perhaps spending most of their time in their room; they may become preoccupied with sexual issues (although parents may not be aware of this preoccupation); they may become "paranoid," convinced that someone or some group is out to get them or is controlling their behavior; or they may begin acting "crazy," seeing things that aren't there or hearing voices that don't exist. If a teenager begins to show these or any combination of these behaviors, parents will want to consult a mental health professional immediately. The relationship between psychosis and adolescence can be confusing to parents and professionals alike. (As one psychiatrist put it, "All adolescents are crazy.") There is a good chance that teenagers who show extreme behaviors of the sort described above may not necessarily be psychotic at all, or if they are, that they will recover fairly quickly from the psychotic episode. In any event, immediate consultation with a mental health facility is necessary.

MANIC-DEPRESSION

"Manic-depression" really refers to two types of disorders; sometimes they occur together, sometimes separately. *Mania* is excessive, disorganized activity. It may include talking compulsively, performing certain activities (such as cleaning or writing) for hours and hours, or such extreme behaviors as running out of the house naked. Parents should realize that teenagers typically, and quite normally, show excessive activity and that this activity is frequently poorly organized, but mania is rather easily distinguished from these normal behaviors. In mania, the person goes on with the activity to a state of exhaustion—and even then still keeps going. For example, manic talkers may talk until their throats are parched and they lose their voice, but still keep talking. In addition, the talking is usually bizarre—for example, talking in rhymes or leaping from thought to thought without making any connections. The parent confronted with a manic teenager will usually recognize in short order that something is very wrong. Obviously, this condition dictates immediate consultation with a mental health facility.

Depression in teenagers is like depression in adults: it can be a normal, if unpleasant, part of life, or it can become so severe that the person cannot live a normal life. Parents of adolescents learn to recognize their child's low spirits, or moodiness, and frequently can help the child to cheer up. In the case of a severe depression, however, efforts to help the child cheer up are to little avail. The child becomes withdrawn, morose, brooding, stops interacting with others, may talk about how "bad" he or she is, may indicate suicidal thoughts, and may have trouble eating, sleeping, and/or having bowel movements. If parents become concerned that their adolescent is more than normally depressed, they should consult a mental health facility immediately. If the depression turns out to be a "normal" one, requiring no outside assistance, then everyone can be relieved and feel better about it. If, however, the depression is a severe one, then the adolescent will be in need of assistance from mental health professionals.

Emotional Disturbances

Just as depression can be mild or severe, so other emotional disturbances that occur during adolescence can be temporary problems that do not require professional assistance, or they can be more severe, persisting problems that would benefit from professional help. Frequently, emotional disturbances will be reflected in teenagers' behavior; some behaviors often associated with emotional problems are discussed below. In other instances, no such specific problem behavior will come to the parent's attention. Instead, they become aware that their child is emotionally troubled. Some examples of adolescent emotional problems include: depression (see discussion above); excessive anxiety about performance in school, sports, and/or social interactions; intense hostility towards other people; extreme fearfulness about something that is not frightening to others. If emotional difficulties are severe and continuing, parents would be well advised to seek professional help for their teenager.

Behavior Problems

EATING

Peculiar eating habits (peculiar, that is, to adults) are frequently a normal aspect of adolescence. There are, however, three types of disturbed eating patterns that occur in adolescence and call for attention from parents. One type is the poor eating that, as described previously, can be part of a depression. Another is called *anorexia nervosa,* a condition in which the teenager stops eating and begins to lose weight to an excessive degree. Anorexia nervosa typically occurs in females and may come about following a diet. The teenage girl may feel she is overweight and may (quite reasonably) begin to diet to lose weight. In a case of anorexia nervosa, however, the teenager does not stop dieting after the desired amount of weight has been lost, but keeps on until she becomes severely emaciated, If parents feel that their child has lost too much weight, they should check with a physician; there can be any number of physical problems that lead to excessive weight loss. If there is no organic problem and the physician believes that anorexia nervosa may be present, a mental health professional should be consulted.

The third type of eating problem that can arise in adolescence is overeating leading to excessive weight gain. Obesity can be a severe problem for teenagers, frequently interfering with their social relationships with peers. Furthermore, as many adults know, overeating is a behavior that is very hard to change once you have become accustomed to it. It is, therefore, very important that parents not overlook a teenager's overeating. Sometimes overeating can be reduced by the parents and child working together without professional help; simple changes in family habits, such as not buying and keeping lots of sweets in the house, can sometimes work wonders. If such simple remedies fail, however, the parent should have the teenager examined by a physician. The physician should be able to indicate how much the child is overweight and whether there is an underlying physical disorder. If the child is significantly overweight and there is no underlying physical disorder present, the physician should help the parents and child construct a weight-loss diet that will ensure that the child has adequate nutrition with fewer calories. If this direct approach fails (which is not unusual) and the child does not lose weight, or continues to gain weight, the parents should consider consulting a mental health professional. This professional can provide the child and family with more extensive changes in their behavior patterns that may help the child in dieting and/or may explore with the child possible emotional problems that contribute to the child's eating behavior.

SLEEPING

Adolescents frequently have sleeping patterns that seem peculiar to adults but that are quite normal for themselves. If, however, the adolescent is bothered by his or her sleep pattern, or if the problem is obviously severe (such as not sleeping for several days), then a physician should be consulted. If no physical problem is found, then it is possible that the sleeping difficulty reflects some kind of emotional problem. In such instances, consultation with a mental health professional is recommended.

AGGRESSION

The overly aggressive teenager is cause for concern. For one thing, teenagers are almost adults physically; too much aggression can lead to actual physical harm to others. Furthermore, the overly aggressive teenager may come into contact with the police and/or the courts, a certainly unpleasant experience that can be the prelude to chronic delinquency. Parents who fear that their teenager is too aggressive should not try to hide their fears from themselves, thus waiting until it becomes far more difficult to help the child. The first response to such a fear should be to discuss the problem with the teenager and try to work out a solution between parent and child. If this does not appear to solve the problem, the parent should consult the child's principal and teachers to see if the aggression observed at home is found at school. (Sometimes, of course, there is aggression at school that teachers bring to the attention of parents who do not observe it at home.) If excessive aggression continues in *either* the home or the school, then consultation with a mental health facility should be sought.

TIMIDITY

It has been noted that social withdrawal can be a symptom of severe problems such as schizophrenia or depression. On the other hand, social withdrawal and avoidance of social interaction can reflect less severe problems such as excessive timidity, shyness, and feelings of social awkwardness These less severe problems can, however, be a cause for concern. Social relations are very important during adolescence, and the lack of good relations with others can make for a very sad adolescence and, in some cases, a lonely adulthood. If parents believe that their child is excessively timid and missing out on the benefits of good social relations with peers, the parents should consult a mental health professional.

SEXUAL PROBLEMS

The teenage years are the years of sexual development, both physically and socially. Many parents have difficulty discussing sexual matters with their child. If this is true, then these parents should make sure that the child has an opportunity to talk over sexual concerns with some other trusted and respected adult (such as a minister or physician). Also, parents may find books that helpfully discuss sexual matters, and they can make these available to the child. In addition, many schools now offer sex-education classes. No matter what the source of learning, what is important is that the teenager be given access to a calm, mature perspective on sex. Virtually all teenagers will learn about sex from their peers, but this learning is often terribly distorted and can lead to biased and misinformed ideas about sex that will hinder more than help the child's development. However they choose to do it, parents have an obligation to help their child learn about sexual functioning.

Most children, of course, manage to learn enough about sex to get through adolescence relatively unscathed. But some children have sexual problems in adolescence. Sometimes these problems take the form of early, precocious, and harmful engagement in sex, sometimes accompanied by an unwanted pregnancy; sometimes the opposite occurs and the child becomes excessively fearful about sex. In the case of either extreme, the parent may want to consider bringing in someone else to help the child—and parent—cope better with the child's sexuality. This outside help can be, again, any trusted adult, such as a minister or physician, who is able to communicate well with both parents and child, or it may be a mental health professional who has been specially trained to discuss sexual matters in an objective manner. Whoever is consulted, this person can be of immense assistance in bridging the gap between parent and child over sexual issues. And such a person can often prevent the continuation of sexual problems that without some assistance can have very unwelcome outcomes, ranging from frantic, unhappy promiscuity to sexual frigidity or impotence.

DRUG-RELATED PROBLEMS

Our era seems to be a time of great concern about drug use by adolescents. In actuality, of course, teenagers have always experimented with drugs of one sort or the other. For my generation, it happened to be alcohol and tobacco; for the present generation, marijuana, most notably, has been added to the list. Parents need to consider carefully the whole issue of drug taking, without jumping to unnecessarily anxious conclusions. In order to assist in this consideration, this section shall describe the immediate and long-range harmful consequences of a variety of drugs. While this description will be brief and limited to only some of the drugs that parents may be concerned about their children taking, it is hoped that it will provide an indication of what is known about certain drugs and the kind of information that might be discussed between parent and child.

First, there is the issue of immediate harm. Tobacco produces relatively little immediate damage. Marijuana and alcohol can have immediate harmful consequences because they can lead to behavior that should not be engaged in when intoxicated or "stoned" (such as driving), but they probably cause little immediate physical damage in and of themselves. Marijuana, of course, as long as it is illegal, can lead to legal problems for the person who smokes it. Amphetamines ("uppers"), barbiturates ("downers"), and cocaine are powerful drugs and can have immediate harmful effects (such as gross impairment of thinking) if taken in excess. The immediate harmful effects of heroin are a matter of controversy; there is, for example, no conclusive evidence that the deaths occurring in association with taking heroin are, in fact, caused by the heroin alone. LSD can, apparently, have immediately harmful effects for some people: it has been reported to have elicited extremely unpleasant experiences and psychotic behavior. Unprescribed taking of all of the above drugs, from amphetamines to LSD, is illegal and can have harmful legal consequences. One "legal" drug (because it is not marketed as a drug) that can have very dangerous immediate consequences is glue. Glue sniffing (or sniffing of any other toxic volatile substance such as gasoline, lighter fluid, paint thinner, and aerosol propellants) is probably the single most dangerous form of drug use and is the most frequent type of drug use during the ages from six to fourteen. The immediate harmful consequences of glue sniffing can range from loss of consciousness to death.

In addition to the immediate effects of drugs, parents must consider the long-range effects, both physical and psychological. Excessive tobacco use is associated with lung cancer and emphysema. Excessive use of alcohol is associated with damage to physical health (such as cirrhosis of the liver) as well as with behavior that can be damaging to the person's psychological, social, and financial well-being. Withdrawal from intensive alcohol use can be quite dangerous, sometimes involving convulsions and/or death. The results of excessive marijuana smoking are not well understood. Some investigators have suggested that excessive marijuana smoking causes a decline of sexual activity and social interest, but the official report of the National Commission on Marijuana and Drug Abuse (1972) does not support this conclusion. As far as is currently known, low levels of consumption of tobacco, alcohol, and marijuana do not have any psychologically harmful consequences. Barbiturates and heroin are addictive drugs; there is dispute about whether amphetamines and cocaine produce physiological addiction. Of this group of drugs, barbiturates are by far the most dangerous in terms of withdrawal; withdrawal may lead to convulsions and/or death. Long-term use of great amounts of amphetamines is accompanied by erratic and unstable behavior. Some people believe that long-term use of *any* level of cocaine and heroin is dangerous; others have argued that long-term use of low levels is not harmful. It is still a matter of controversy about how painful it is to terminate the taking of heroin after becoming addicted. It is clear that if a pregnant woman is addicted to heroin, her child will be born addicted to the drug and will need immediate medical care. Long-term effects of LSD are not well understood. Some people report positive effects (such as heightened creativity); others have had psychotic reactions. The exact relationship of the drug to either of these effects is not known. Glue sniffing is, of course, even more dangerous when used repeatedly. A person's chances of brain damage or death increase greatly with repeated usage.

It is hoped that this brief summary will provide parents with some basic information about drugs. Many parents may prefer that their children not take any of the above drugs, and some children will grow into adulthood without taking any of them. Other children will sample some of the more socially acceptable drugs such as tobacco and alcohol (and, increasingly, marijuana) without forming any long-term dependency on them. Others will become highly involved with a variety of drugs. The first step in preventing drug problems in children is to make sure children have adequate information about drugs. Parents must make sure that their children—and, hopefully, themselves as well—are exposed to the most *accurate* information about drugs that is available. "Scare tactics" may not only fail to prevent drug use, but may also increase the likelihood of adverse psychological reactions when a drug is taken.

Parents and children should discuss drugs and drug taking with each other. These discussions are important to clarify the confusion that often results when children hear their parents say, "Don't take any drugs," but observe their parents smoking cigarettes, drinking alcohol, and taking sleeping pills. Clearly, such parents are not avoiding all drugs; they are making distinctions among drugs, and these distinctions should be discussed with their children. These discussions may also serve to highlight parental responsibility for children's drug use. For example, it has been found that the best predictor of child drug use is parental drug use. As a result of discussions with their children, parents as well as children may decide to change their drug use.

If information and parent-child discussion are made available to the child, but the parent still believes that the child has a drug problem—that is, that the child is taking too much of a drug, is using a harmful drug (no matter what the amount), or is courting legal disaster by using an illegal drug—then parents may want to consider obtaining some sort of drug counseling for the child. There are drug-counseling centers in most communities; typically these centers are supervised by mental health professionals. The parent can go with the child to such a center or attempt to have the child go on his or her own if the child prefers. Also, the parent can go to a mental health facility for either counseling there or referral to a drug-counseling center.

In any case, the troubled parent should make contact in some way with someone qualified to advise about drugs. As with other problems we have discussed, the apparent drug problem *may* be a problem for the child — *or* the problem may be that the parent has unrealistic expectations or inaccurate beliefs. Whatever the case, drug taking *can* be very dangerous indeed, and parents should feel free to seek help when they are troubled.

Communication Disorders

STUTTERING

It was noted previously that most children who stutter do not continue to do so as they grow older. However, for those children who do continue to stutter, adolescence can be a difficult time. Stuttering can be an embarrassing, socially awkward behavior that disrupts relationships with peers. If parents have a teenager who stutters, they can obtain assistance for the teenager's speech problem from a speech clinic. If, in addition to the speech problem, the teenager appears to have trouble getting along with peers and making friends, parents should consider consulting a mental health facility.

TRAUMATIC INJURY TO THE BRAIN

One type of severe language difficulty that can occur during adolescence involves traumatic damage to the brain.[3] Adolescents who suffer severe head injuries may have language difficulties that persist long after their physical recovery. A child confronted with such problems will be offered rehabilitative language training that will be recommended and, usually, arranged by the medical personnel involved. In addition, however, there

---

[3] Traumatic injury to the brain can occur to children of any age, and so most of the comments in this section are applicable to any age group. Language impairment as a result of traumatic brain damage is especially significant for adolescents because other types of communication problems are usually recognized at earlier ages, and the social and emotional consequences of sudden language impairment can be especially disturbing for teenagers.

can be important psychological aspects to consider. It is a terrible experience for a teenager to be fine one day, have an accident, and then wake up with a severe language problem. Trying to cope with this experience can lead to emotional and behavioral problems. As is the case with physically handicapped children, the people who work with the brain-damaged child will usually be able to help the child through emotional or behavior problems. If, however, these problems persist or become more severe, the parent should think about consulting a mental health professional.

Physically Handicapped Children

Adolescence is a particularly frustrating time for the physically handicapped. At this time, physique becomes especially important as adolescents become more aware of their potential sexuality. Also, peer groups tend to be more powerful, either as a source of distress or support, than they were at younger ages. The adolescent with a typical physique may suffer from emotional and/or behavioral problems as a direct result of these adolescent experiences. If such problems do arise, the parent can obtain help for the child from a mental health facility.

COLLECTING INFORMATION: HOW IT CAN HELP PARENTS AND PROFESSIONALS

"The horror of that moment," the King went on, "I shall never, *never* forget!"
"You will, though," the Queen said, "if you don't make a memorandum of it."

Through the Looking-Glass

Parents may wonder about what information they should collect before going to a mental health professional. In the case of a physical problem, parents are used to collecting information. For example, if a parent is concerned that a child has a fever, the parent typically takes the child's temperature before consulting the pediatrician. This information serves to help parents decide whether or not to consult a physician and, when it is reported to the physician, can help the physician administer prompt treatment. Similarly, in the case of consulting a mental health professional, it can be of invaluable assistance to both parent and professional if the parent has taken good notes on the child's behavior.

What are "good" notes? Let us consider a specific problem, such as a child's hitting other children (or staying in his or her room for long periods of time, or throwing temper tantrums). In such instances, the parent can jot down *when* the behavior occurred, *where* it occurred, *how long* it lasted, and *what happened as a result* of the behavior. The parent can also note what steps have already been taken to deal with the problem and the consequences of these actions. An example of this type of note taking is given below.

PROBLEM: JOHNNY'S HITTING OTHER CHILDREN

Johnny hit Sally, who had taken his toy away from him.

When: 11:00 A.M., Mon., April 18, 1977.

Where: Playground.

Duration: Hit her twice; just a few minutes.

Afterward: Sally cried; Johnny got the toy.

What I did: Went over and told Johnny not to hit Sally. Told Sally not to take Johnny's toys away from him.

Afterward: Sally tried to take Johnny's toy again; I stopped her. No hitting.

Johnny hit Billy, who was playing with his own (Billy's) toy.

When: 11:15 A.M., Tues., May 17, 1977.

Where: Playgroung.

Duration: Hit Billy four times; few minutes.

Afterward: Billy cried; Johnny got Billy's toy.

What I did: Went over and told Johnny not to hit Billy or take his toy away. Gave Billy his toy back.

Afterward: Johnny hit Billy again.

Notes such as these can be very useful to a mental health professional. They also can help the parent decide how severe the problem is. If, for example, Johnny's behavior in the examples above occurred only once a month and Johnny was three years old, most parents wouldn't be concerned. If, on the other hand, Johnny's behavior occurred much more frequently or Johnny was much older, or if the behavior was much more intense, then his parents might well be concerned.

But what if the problem isn't so specific? What if it is, for example, that Judy feels depressed — but she doesn't stay in her room, doesn't have sleeping problems, doesn't stop dressing well, or have any other clear behavior difficulties? In this case, the parents are not concerned about any one specific behavior, but about Judy's feelings and her general behavior. It is quite possible to take notes about such concerns. The parents can jot down their impressions of how Judy *used to be* and how she has *changed*. They can also try to recollect *when* the change occurred, *what else was happening* in Judy's life when it occurred, and *what they and others have done* to try to help Judy and with what *results*. These notes, just as ones on more specific behaviors, can serve the double function of helping parents get their thoughts in order as they decide whether to consult a mental health facility about Judy's depression and of assisting the mental health professional, if consulted, to help Judy more promptly and effectively.

> "Would you tell me, please, which way I ought to go from here?" "That depends a good deal on where you want to get to," said the Cat.
>
> *Alice's Adventures in Wonderland*

How Do I Find a Mental Health Facility?

CHAPTER 3

GETTING PAST THE EMOTIONAL BARRIERS

Even when parents have decided that they want to consult a mental health professional about their child, there are two major obstacles to their actually obtaining this assistance. The first obstacle is a psychological one. (The second—finding the right kind of facility—is discussed in the next section.)

Parents have all kinds of feelings that can lead them to avoid contacting a mental health facility. Some parents worry that they will look silly if their child turns out not to need any kind of mental health care. Others worry that going to a mental health facility means they have failed as parents. Others worry that going to a mental health facility means that they or their child must be "crazy"—or at least will be considered "crazy" by other people. All of these concerns can be felt very strongly and can serve as real barriers, preventing parents who think they should go to a mental health facility from ever actually getting there. Let us discuss each of these feelings and suggest some ways for parents to cope with them.

First, there is the worry about looking silly if what the parents thought was a problem turns out not to be a problem at all. Parents don't have this concern only about mental health facilities; they can also worry about looking silly when they take their child to the pediatrician or dentist or any other expert. It is true, of course, that you do not want to run off to an expert every time any little difficulty occurs. Parents don't consult their pediatrician every time their child has the sniffles, nor their dentist every time a baby tooth falls out. Similarly, parents would not want to consult a mental health professional every time their child has a temper tantrum.

But if a parent has carefully considered a problem and has decided that expert assistance is needed, then the parent should feel confident about consulting the expert. If it turns out that the mental (or physical or dental) health problem is, in fact, not a problem, then the parent should feel relieved and should certainly not feel silly. It is *always* better to find that a suspected problem isn't really a problem after all — or isn't as serious as one though — than to run the risk of letting a real problem go unattended. In terms of their child's mental health, parents should never feel embarrassed about going to a mental health facility and finding out that the child's behavior is actually quite normal and psychologically healthy. The parent in this situation should feel relieved and should feel good about being a concerned and conscientious parent who gets expert advice when it is needed. Experts can serve to relieve worries as much as to indicate that there really is a problem to be worried about.

Another concern that parents have is that going to a mental health facility means that they have failed as parents. This concern is understandable. It is true that parents first try to solve problems on their own, and usually only go to someone else when they are unable to solve the problem. Parents should, however, try to put this concern into perspective. For example, is the parent a failure who consults a pediatrician when the child has a high fever? Obviously not. Similarly in regard to children's mental health, the successful parent is the one who obtains expert advice when it is needed. Recognizing that a difficult problem needs assistance is *not* the mark of failure as a parent; obtaining this assistance *is* an expression of love for the child.

What, then, about the concern about seeming to be "crazy"? While there has been tremendous progress in our attitudes about mental health problems, it is still true that obtaining mental health care is regarded by some as a shameful sort of thing that only "crazy" people need to do. This attitude is based on fear and lack of knowledge about mental health problems and their treatment. Once people find out about what sorts of things are involved in mental health problems and what sorts of things mental health professionals really do, such irrational attitudes usually change a great deal. Parents who recognize such attitudes in themselves can best cope with these attitudes by obtaining more information. It is hoped, for example, that any parent who reads this book will begin to develop a more informed and thus less fearful attitude about mental health problems. As for other people, parents can try to educate them — have them read this or some other informative book on mental health care — but in some cases, parents may have to ignore the opinions of others and simply go ahead with what they think is right and beneficial for their child and themselves. Parents have their first obligations to their child and to themselves; they are not responsible for the fearful and irrational attitudes of others.

GETTING PAST THE PRACTICAL BARRIERS

Once parents have decided that they wish to consult a mental health facility and have overcome any emotional barriers to doing so, there is still the very real difficulty of finding such a place. In finding a mental health facility, the major question to ask is what *kind* of facility is appropriate for the specific child's specific problem. The following guidelines are offered to assist in answering this question.

Special Needs

Is it an emergency situation? If the parent is confronted with an emergency situation (for example, a suicide attempt by the child), the best place to go for immediate help is the emergency room of the nearest hospital. The personnel there can provide any physical treatment that may be needed (from stitches to tranquilizers); they can hospitalize the child if this is necessary; and they can put the parent in contact with mental health personnel either at that hospital or at some nearby facility. A psychological emergency should be treated just as any other emergency; one should go to the place prepared to deliver emergency care, and that generally is the emergency room of the nearest hospital.

Another alternative available in some communities is a "crisis center" or "hotline." These are telephone answering centers where trained personnel are continually on call to help people deal with crisis situations. The personnel at these centers can talk the problem over with parents and can also refer them to a specific mental health facility if this is needed. In order to find out if a "hotline" is available in a community and, if it is, to obtain the number, one need only call the local information operator and ask. A general rule of thumb in regard to hotlines versus emergency rooms is that the emergency room is to be preferred if there is any physical danger to the child or to the people around him or her. If there is no actual physical danger, but there is an intense, hard-to-handle psychological problem, the hotline may be more helpful.

Additional resources that can be utilized in an emergency situation include physicians; ministers, priests, or rabbis; and the police. A psychological emergency with one's child is no time to be shy or feel embarrassed. Parents should get the quickest help they can to deal with the immediate situation. Decisions about what kind of continuing help might be needed can be made later when the situation has calmed down.

Is there the possibility that a physical problem is involved? In the discussion in Chapter 2 it was noted, especially in regard to preschoolers, that many pshchological problems may involve physical problems as well. If the parent thinks the apparent psychological problem may also involve a physical problem, the best first consultation is, as noted, with the child's pediatrician.

Is there the possibility that a school problem is involved? Again, the discussion in Chapter 2 noted those occasions upon which the best first consultation may be with the child's teacher and principal. It was also noted that school psychologists, if they are available, can provide important assistance.

People such as teachers and pediatricians can refer the parent to mental health facilities. The parent can then either follow up these referrals or, if preferred, go to mental health facilities other than those recommended. The choice probably will rest on how much confidence the parent has in the teacher or pediatrician. If a parent has a good relationship with a teacher or pediatrician and respects this person, the parent should follow this person's advice; teachers and pediatricians are familiar with the resources in the community and can serve to direct the parent to the mental health facility that is likely to provide the best service. It should be reemphasized, however, that (1) the parent retains the final decision, *and* (2) if a consulted teacher or pediatrician does not refer the parent to a mental health facility, but the parent wishes to consult one anyway, the parent can do so on his or her own. Other professionals who might be consulted for a specific problem, but who can also make referrals to mental health facilities, include: speech and language specialists (often called speech therapists), physical therapists, nurses, and social workers.

Is the child of preschool age? Most preschool children who need psychological assistance also need educational and perhaps medical assistance. It is thus most helpful if young children are initially evaluated by a team of professionals, including, for example, a pediatrician, a psychologist, a speech and language specialist, and an educational consultant. These types of multifaceted evaluations are available at developmental evaluation clinics found in many major medical centers. It may be well worth the effort and expense for a parent who has concerns about a preschool child to find out from a pediatrician where the nearest developmental evaluation clinic is located, and, if at all possible, arrange to take the child there for the initial evaluation. The pediatrician can help make these arrangements, or the parent can call or write the nearest clinic for an appointment. If the nearest such clinic is just too far away and is not a feasible alternative, the parent should ask the pediatrician about the nearest pediatrics department in a general hospital where there is a pediatric psychologist. An evaluation by this pediatrics department can thus include a psychological assessment as well as a physical examination. Again, an appointment can be arranged by the pediatrician or by the parent.

A SURVEY OF TYPES OF MENTAL HEALTH FACILITIES

If none of the above specific questions is relevant for a particular child, then the parent will want to contact one of the following types of mental health facilities. In most communities, several types of facilities are available. The following survey describes a number of features that parents may wish to consider when they decide which type of facility would be best for them and their child.

Private Practitioners

In most communities, there are mental health professionals engaged in private practice. These professionals are self-employed, rather than working for a clinic or hospital. The majority of private practitioners are psychiatrists, psychologists, and social workers. The names, addresses, and phone numbers of private practitioners in a community can be found in the yellow pages of the phone book under a general heading like Physicians and Surgeons—Doctors of Medicine; Psychologists; and Social Workers. For physicians, their specialty area is usually indicated in some way; all psychiatrists (sometimes termed "neuropsychiatrists") may be grouped together or there may be an alphabetical name listing that includes the field of specialization.

In going to a private practitioner, a few matters must be kept in mind. First, you want to make sure you see a qualified person. Chapter 4 describes the training, experience, and licensing/certification that psychiatrists, psychologists, and social workers need to have in order to be qualified to work with clients. Additionally, parents should make sure that the practitioner has special expertise in working with children; frequently, such expertise is designated in the phone book listing of the practitioner (for example, "Child psychiatry," "Child psychology").

In considering a private practitioner, parents can ask the professional about his or her training, experience, and licensing/certification to see if the practitioner has completed the minimum necessary requirements. Indeed, many private practitioners have their diplomas displayed on the walls of their offices where their clients can see them. If it is not clear from this information whether or not the professional has special expertise in working with children, parents should ask the practitioner about this. Being qualified in terms of training, experience, licensing/certification, and specialization in childhood problems does not guarantee that any given private practitioner is excellent at what he or she does. When professionals are qualified in the above ways, it does guarantee that they have met a minimum level of competence in fulfilling the requirements of their profession.

Another matter to be kept in mind about seeing a private practitioner is the expense. Most parents need to find out rather quickly how much the practitioner charges and how much total expense is likely to be incurred in helping their child. Private practitioners may be unable to give an exact amount of anticipated expense, but they should be able to give a reasonable estimate. Parents also need to check with their insurance company to see how much of this expense will be covered by insurance (see Chapter 9). In general, private practitioners are rather expensive.

Finally, it is most helpful if parents can find out about a particular practitioner's reputation. If there is a friend or relative who has had contact with the private practitioner, this person's opinion can be helpful. Useful information can also come from people who have lived in the community a number of years, who are in a position to know the reputation of professionals in the community, and whose judgment the parent respects. Such people include ministers, priests, and rabbis; other physicians; social workers; teachers; and lawyers. Also, in some communities there are local chapters of parents' and citizens' groups that work in assisting children with specific types of problems. If parents believe their child may have one of these specific problems, the local chapter can help find out about the practitioner's reputation (see p. 161 for information on how to find out about such groups). Regardless of who is consulted on this issue, parents will feel much better about going to a private practitioner who has been recommended by someone known and respected by the parents.

Child Guidance Clinics

Child guidance clinics are specifically designed to work with children and families on mental health problems. If one is available in a community, it will be listed in the phone book, in the white pages under city or county agencies and in the yellow pages under (mental) health agencies. Usually at least some of the staff at a child guidance clinic are associated with a local hospital. This association usually guarantees that the staff at the clinic meet the minimum qualifications of training and experience noted above. If no such association exists, parents should inquire about the qualifications of the staff.

Many child guidance clinics provide training for mental health professionals, and thus some of the staff members are likely to be psychiatrists, psychologists, or social workers in training. Parents should be aware of both the advantages and disadvantages of working with a mental health professional who is still being trained. The obvious disadvantage is that the trainee is not as experienced as the fully qualified professional. This is not necessarily a serious disadvantage if the trainee is being carefully supervised by a fully qualified person at the clinic. When a parent is working with a trainee, it is the parent's right to inquire about the trainee's supervision so that the parent may have confidence that the trainee's work reflects both his or her own judgment and the approval of that judgment by a more experienced person. Almost all trainees would prefer that parents inquire about this so that their questions can be answered and their confidence gained, rather than for parents to be concerned about this, and perhaps not fully trust the trainee, but never bring it up. The advantage to working with a trainee is that not infrequently trainees are very enthusiastic and involved in their work, and will go to a great deal of trouble to help their clients. Also, since they are receiving training, the trainees may be seeing fewer clients than full professionals would and have more time to spend in helping each one. Additionally, trainees may be more familiar with current advances in the field than the fully qualified professionals who received their training a number of years ago.

Most child guidance clinics operate on a "sliding scale" for fees. This means that parents will have to inform the clinic of their income (this information, of course, to be kept in strictest confidence), and the clinic will set the fee in accordance with this income: parents with a large income will be charged more than parents with a small income for the same services. Most child guidance clinics could not afford to operate on the basis of the fees they charge; they receive additional support from community organizations (such as the United Fund and/or a local hospital). Parents need to inquire about the clinic's fee scale and to check on how much their insurance will cover (see Chapter 9); clinics typically have someone to help them do this.

Finally, the suggestions made above about determining reputation apply to clinics as well as to private practitioners. Parents can talk with people who are in a position to know about or who have had contact with the clinic. Since the clinic is a community institution, it will usually be easier to find out about a clinic than to find out about a private practitioner.

Community Mental Health Centers

Community mental health centers are similar in some ways to child guidance clinics except that while the clients of child guidance clinics are children (usually up to age sixteen or eighteen), the clients of community mental health centers are usually adults. Thus, the first thing parents need to find out about a community mental health center is whether that facility will see children of their child's age. They can do this by calling or visiting the center; center's phone numbers and addresses are listed in the phone book in the same ways as those of child guidance clinics. If the child is an adolescent, the center probably will see the child; if the child is younger, the center may not. If the center does agree to see an adolescent or child, the parent should inquire whether there is someone on the staff who works especially with children and ask to see that person. If the community mental health center does not have someone experienced in working with children, or if the center will not see a younger child, the parent should ask to be referred to local agencies where there are child specialists.

Community mental health centers are funded by local government agencies and often by the federal government as well. This means that fees are likely to be on a sliding scale (see Chapter 9). It also means that the parent usually can be assured that the staff will have met minimum qualifications of training and experience. Additionally, there may be trainees at the center, and the previous discussion of trainees also applies here. Finally, parents should also check out the reputation of the center in the community.

Hospital Departments of Psychiatry

Many hospitals have departments of psychiatry. In considering a hospital, parents need to call and find out if there is a department of psychiatry and, if so, whether the department will see children of their child's age. Guidelines concerning what to do if they will or will not are the same as those for community mental health centers. Hospitals may or may not charge on a sliding scale, and parents need to inquire about this and about insurance (see Chapter 9). As long as the hospital is an established one in the community, the staff usually will have met minimum qualifications of training and experience. Frequently, there are trainees working at the hospital, and previous remarks concerning trainees are also applicable here. Finally, parents should investigate the reputation of the specific department of psychiatry (not just the reputation of the hospital) in the community.

Veterans Administration Hospitals

Veterans Administration hospitals provide mental health services for those veterans meeting the V.A.'s eligibility standards. Until quite recently, most mental health services were provided only for the veteran and not for the veteran's family. Lately, some V.A. hospitals have become interested in providing family-oriented mental health services. Thus, some of them are now able to provide mental health services for children. Parents who are eligible for and interested in obtaining V.A. mental health services should contact their local V.A.—the phone number can be found in the white pages of the phone book under "United States Government—Veterans Administration." In contacting the V.A., parents should inquire if the V.A. hospital will see children of their child's age. Guidelines concerning what to do if the V.A. will or will not see their child are the same as those given for community mental health centers. Standards for the professional qualifications of V.A. hospital staff are set by the federal government, and thus parents do not need to be concerned about the staff's having met minimum qualifications of training and experience. Frequently, there are trainees working at the hospital, and previous remarks concerning trainees are also applicable here. And, once again, parents should investigate the community reputation of the specific department of psychiatry or psychology that would see their child.

Group Homes

It has become increasingly evident to mental health professionals that many people need residential facilities without necessarily needing hospitalization. This recognition has led to the establishment of group homes in many communities. There are a variety of types of group homes: some provide residence facilities for people who have been hospitalized previously; some are for mentally retarded individuals; some are for people who have been released from prison; some are for people with drug usage difficulties; and some are for adolescents who have difficulties living at home. To find out if there is a group home in the community and if there is a specific type of group home that might meet the specific needs of one's child, a parent should call the local community mental health center. Typically, group homes accept people only on the basis of a referral, and frequently the local community mental health center makes these referalls.

State Hospitals

State hospitals, either psychiatric or for the mentally retarded, frequently will not see clients on an outpatient basis; that is, they typically only work with clients hospitalized in their institution. Additionally, many state hospitals will only consider for hospitalization those clients who have been referred to them from other agencies. If parents are concerned that their child may need to be hospitalized, they can consult any of the other mental health facilities described in this summary. They can also call a state hospital (number listed in the phone book of the community in which the state hospital is located, or may be obtained from any mental health professional) and ask whether or not a referral for hospitalization is necessary and, if so, where it is recommended that evaluations and referrals be obtained.

Private Residence Facilities

There are a number of facilities that provide resident care for children with mental health problems. These facilities differ from state hospitals in that payment for care is on a private basis (generally through insurance) rather than from public sources of funds (see Chapter 9 for further discussion of the differences between public and private funding). Private residence facilities for children are frequently called "schools for the emotionally disturbed." These facilities vary widely in whether they see outpatients as well as inpatients and in whether they require that clients be referred to them by other agencies. If a parent is interested in any specific private residence facility, the best approach is to call the facility and ask about its policies.

This concludes our survey of possible mental health facilities that parents may have available to them. There are some variations that have not been discussed (for example, a clinic made up of private practitioners, the characteristics of such a clinic usually being quite similar to those described above for individual private practitioners), but in general our survey has covered the most typical ones. There are, of course, many more questions that a parent will have about mental health facilities, and these will be covered in other chapters. For now, this survey should serve to indicate the range of possible facilities available and to provide an indication of the sort of information a parent can obtain in making a decision to go to one place rather than to another.

> "What's the use of their having names," the Gnat said, "if they won't answer to them?"
> "No use to *them*," said Alice; "but it's useful to the people that name them, I suppose. If not, why do things have names at all?"
>
> *Through the Looking-Glass*

Who Will I Meet at a Mental Health Facility?

CHAPTER 4

As we have seen, many things must happen before a parent ever arrives at a mental health facility. The parent must become concerned about the child and decide that the advice of a mental health professional is needed. The parent must decide what type of mental health facility would be best for the child, locate this facility, and make an appointment to be seen at this facility. Only after all of this will parent and child actually come into the facility.

One of the most confusing things for many parents when they go to a mental health facility—or even when they make their initial phone contact with the facility—is the large number of people in different professions that they may meet. Many parents do not understand how these professions differ, and they may be confused as to what services they can expect from members of any one profession. It would be helpful for parents if they knew the difference between, for example, a psychiatrist and a psychologist, and didn't have to use valuable time and effort trying to figure out this difference on their own.

This chapter is designed to provide that assistance. Here you will find a brief description of a variety of professionals who work in the mental health field. Their training will be described, as will the activities in which they most typically engage. It should be noted that not all mental health facilities will have all the types of professionals described in this chapter; however, in order to give the most useful information, a wide range of professions that might possibly be found in at least some mental health facilities will be described.

MAJOR MENTAL HEALTH PROFESSIONS

Three professions—psychiatry, psychology, and social work—constitute the major mental health professions. All clinics that offer general mental health services will have at least one of each of these professionals working there, and some members of each of these professions work as private practitioners (see Chapter 3). It used to be fairly easy to know the difference among these three professions in terms of the services each offered: psychiatrists gave treatment; psychologists administered tests and conducted research; social workers interviewed clients about their history and worked with community organizations such as the courts and welfare services. More recently, these easy distinctions have largely broken down. Members of all three professions provide psychological treatment, some members of all three professions conduct research, and, increasingly, all three professions emphasize the importance of working with community organizations. Thus, if you just look at what they do, it can be difficult to tell the difference among psychiatrists, psychologists, and social workers—and, in some facilities, it can be of relatively little importance. On the other hand, members of these three professions do come from quite different training backgrounds, and each profession still has special expertise in certain areas. The sections below will describe each of these three professions in terms of their training and their special skills.

PSYCHIATRISTS

Psychiatrists are college graduates who have completed medical school and received their medical degree (M.D.). They have then completed a residency in psychiatry (usually of three to four years' duration) during which time they have administered psychiatric treatment under the supervision of experienced mental health professionals. Fully qualified psychiatrists have also passed national examinations in their specialty area; psychiatrists who have passed these examinations are called "board-certified."

Psychiatrists are licensed by the state to practice medicine and can prescribe medication. They are qualified to conduct psychological treatment such as psychotherapy or behavior therapy (see Chapters 6 and 7 for discussion of these therapies). A psychiatrist can also administer physical forms of treatment such as medication and electroconvulsive therapy (ECT — see Chapter 6). Psychiatrists are not qualified to administer intelligence or personality tests (see Chapter 6 for description of these tests). Psychiatrists do conduct research into the origin and characteristics of mental health problems, but their training programs do not emphasize research as much as the training programs of psychologists.

Psychoanalysts

In order to become a psychoanalyst, a person must receive training from a psychoanalytic institute. These institutes offer specialized work in Freudian theory and psychoanalytic treatment.[1] Although Freud himself did not believe that a person must have a M.D. degree in order to become a psychoanalyst, many institutes in the United States have required this, and at present most psychoanalysts in this country are M.D.'s who have completed their residency as well as their training at an institute.

PSYCHOLOGISTS

Psychologists as a group represent a diverse collection of interests relating to human behavior. Many psychologists deliver services to clinics, schools, organizations, and individuals; however, a large number pursue academic and research endeavors exclusively. Persons employed as psychologists have completed college and then a graduate school program leading to an M.S. (master of science), M.A. (master of arts), Ph.D. (Doctor

---

[1]Freudian psychoanalysis is a specific approach to the understanding and treatment of psychological problems originated by Sigmund Freud (1856-1939). Major techniques consist of the patient's "free-associating" (that is, stating everything that comes to mind) and the therapist's making "interpretations." See Chapter 6 for further discussion.

of philosophy), or Ed.D. (doctor of education) degree. State regulations and professional organizations are increasingly requiring that those psychologists who deal directly and independently with clients complete a doctoral training program (Ph.D. or Ed.D.), plus a year of postdoctoral work in their specialty area, and pass a state-regulated examination to become certified as qualified psychologists. Psychologists with master's-level training who deliver mental health services should have had at least one year's supervised clinical work, have passed the state-regulated examination, and have a psychiatrist or doctoral-level psychologist available for consultation or supervision.

Psychologists are not qualified to administer medication or other forms of physical treatment. They are qualified to conduct psychological treatment and to assess intellectual and personality functioning through the use of test materials designed for these purposes. By virtue of their graduate school training programs, Ph.D.- and Ed.D.-level psychologists are intensively trained in research methods, and many are actively engaged in conducting research on mental health problems.

SOCIAL WORKERS

Social workers are college graduates who have received training in a graduate school of social work and have had practical experience in a variety of settings. Social workers have received the M.S.W. degree (master of social work), and some social workers, especially those that wish to specialize in teaching and research, have received their doctorate (Ph.D. in social work or related field; or D.S.W., doctors of social work). Social workers are certified by a national examining board, and many states require that social workers engaged in mental health services be licensed to practice by the state.

Social workers are not qualified to prescribe medication, administer physical treatment, or conduct testing of intellectual or personality functioning. Many social workers are qualified to conduct psychological treatment,[2] and some engage in research. Almost all social workers are specially trained to conduct intake interviews in which they find out about the

---

[2] An M.S.W. qualified to conduct psychological treatment will have had at least one year's supervised experience in conducting therapy and, preferably, will have a psychiatrist or doctoral level psychologist or social worker available for supervision or consultation.

"presenting complaint" (what brings a person to the facility) and about the person's general life circumstances (family, job, etc.). Many social workers are also highly skilled in dealing with bureaucratic organizations such as welfare agencies, the court system, and vocational training programs. Social workers who have specialized in mental health care may be called "psychiatric" or "clinical" social workers.

MENTAL HEALTH WORKERS FOUND PRIMARILY IN INPATIENT MENTAL HEALTH FACILITIES

Psychiatrists, psychologists, and social workers are found in mental health facilities that provide outpatient care (that is, where the person receiving treatment lives at home and comes to the facility for treatment) and in those that provide inpatient care (where the person lives at the mental health facility while receiving treatment). The following two types of mental health workers are most typically found only at facilities that provide inpatient care.

Psychiatric Nurses

Nurses are high school graduates who complete a course in nurses' training. Sometimes this training is offered as part of a college degree program, the graduates of this program receiving a B.S. (bachelor of science in nursing) degree. Sometimes nurses receive their training in two- or three-year courses offered by nursing schools that are part of a junior college or hospital; graduates of these programs, who also complete a required number of college credits, receive an associate or diploma degree in nursing. When nurses complete any of these types of training and pass state and national examinations, they are then called registered nurses (RNs) and are professionals certified to administer nursing care. Nurses who have received their B.S. may also go on to further training in nursing at the M.S. (master of science) or Ph.D. (doctor of philosophy in nursing) levels; the latter degrees are more important for administration and teaching than for direct patient care. RNs are qualified to administer medication as ordered by a physician, check a patient's physical status (take blood pressure, temperature, etc.), and administer all patient care ordered by the attending physician. Nurses who are specially trained to deal with psychological problems are called "psychiatric nurses." With supervision by a psychiatrist or psychologist, psychiatric nurses may conduct psychological treatment.

Licensed practical nurses (LPNs) are usually high school graduates who have completed a certified course in practical nursing. LPNs are qualified to administer general patient care as ordered by a physician and as supervised by a RN. In some facilities, LPNs, under the supervision of a psychiatric nurse, may conduct some forms of psychological treatment such as group therapy (see Chapter 6 for description of group therapy).

Psychiatric Aides or Attendants

There are no general rules concerning the education or training received by aides or attendants. Sometimes they are adults who may or may not have completed high school; sometimes they are college students. Usually they have completed a short course of training offered by the facility that employs them. Aides are usually responsible for the routine work necessary to keep an inpatient facility going (making beds, serving food, keeping the ward clean, etc.) Aides are not qualified to prescribe or administer drugs, give physical treatment, administer psychological tests, or conduct psychological treatment. In short, they are not qualified to engage in any of the special services carried on by the professionals described previously in this chapter. Aides are nevertheless very important people in a mental health facility. Typically, aides have more contact with the patients than any of the other mental health professionals. They talk with the patients, help keep them from getting bored (for example, by playing cards with adult inpatients or playing basketball with children), escort them on walks both inside and outside the facility, and in general tend to their personal needs when necessary. A sensitive, helpful aide can make an important positive contribution to an inpatient's treatment program; an insensitive or hostile aide can have a strongly negative effect on such a program.

ALLIED PROFESSIONS

In addition to the various types of occupations in the mental health field described above, there are members of allied professions who do not necessarily specialize in the delivery of mental health care, but who do have skills that can contribute significantly in providing such care.

Physicians

There are a variety of physicians who, although not psychiatrists, can participate in the evaluation and treatment of mental health problems. These physicians (like all physicians) are college graduates who have completed medical school received their M.D. degree. They have all taken a residency in their specialty area and to complete their specialization, will pass national examinations in their specialty area becoming board-certified. All are licensed by the state to practice medicine and prescribe medication. All are qualified to administer various physical treatments relevant to their specialty area.

PEDIATRICIANS

Some pediatricians specialize in pediatric problems that involve psychological factors, such as mental retardation and obesity. The majority of pediatricians, however, are involved in delivering general care to children. As indicated in Chapter 2, there are many psychological problems during childhood where the first person to be consulted is a pediatrician.

NEUROLOGISTS

Neurologists are consulted whenever there is a concern that a psychological problem may involve some sort of damage to the nervous system.

REHABILITATION PHYSICIANS

Rehabilitation physicians work with people who have suffered some significant loss in their physical functioning (for example, have had damage to their spinal cord, have suffered a stroke, have lost a limb) and need assistance in resuming an active daily life. Rehabilitation physicians are responsible for the general rehabilitative program designed to help the patient resume an active life, and frequently work with psychologists and psychiatrists to provide a program that addresses the patient's psychological as well as physical rehabilitation. Psychologists who specialize in rehabilitation are called rehabilitation psychologists.

Speech and Language Specialists

A speech and language specialist is a college graduate who has received graduate training in audiology and/or speech pathology. Such specialists may have a M.A. (master of arts) or Ph.D. (doctor of philosophy in speech pathology) degree. A speech and language specialist is qualified to assess a person's ability to comprehend and use verbal language and to produce speech. The speech and language specialist helps design and administer treatment programs to improve speech and language skills. This assessment and planning is usually done in conjunction with an audiologist, who assesses the person's ability to hear. Chapter 2 described the importance of speech and language specialists in working with children who have communication problems.

Educational Consultants

An educational consultant is a college graduate who typically has received additional training in special education (the education of handicapped and/or emotionally disturbed children). Usually an educational consultant has an M.A., although some may have completed a Ed.D. program. Many educational consultants have had extensive teaching experience. Educational consultants can be most valuable in planning an educational program that will best meet the needs of an individual child who has a psychological difficulty.

Occupational Therapists and Physical Therapists

Occupational and physical therapists are college (or master's level) graduates of specialized programs in occupational or physical therapy who have passed a state and/or national certification examination in occupational or physical therapy. Both occupational therapists and physical therapists assess and treat a variety of problems found in areas such as movement and dexterity, visual and/or perceptual development, and self-help skills such as feeding and dressing.

CONCERNING THE "TEAM" APPROACH

One final note needs to be made about the diverse number of professionals who work at a mental health facility. In recent years, a "team" approach to mental health care has become popular. A team approach means that a variety of people from different professions will work with one child or family. This type of approach often makes a good deal of sense, in that many children require a variety of types of professional services in order to receive the best possible mental health care. The team approach can, however, be somewhat confusing to parents who suddenly have to meet a number of different people from different professions. Parents who are working with a team should feel free to ask who the members of the team are and what they *each* will contribute to the evaluation or treatment of the child or family. Parents should also feel free to request that one member of the team act as team coordinator and be available to the prarent for discussing *all* of the team's work. Such coordinators are usually designated in advance for just this purpose, but if they are not, the parent might well ask that such a position be created. By having one person responsible for talking with the parent, parents are spared the ordeal of having to figure out just which professional should be asked which question. With a team coordinator, all questions are addressed to one person who is in a much better position than the parent to consult with other team members if this is necessary in order to answer any specific questions.

> "What do you mean by 'If you really are a Queen'? What right have you to call yourself so? You can't be a Queen, you know, till you've passed the proper examination. And the sooner we begin it, the better."
>
> Through the Looking-Glass

How Will a Mental Health Facility Determine If My Child Needs Treatment?

CHAPTER 5

At this point in our step-by-step sequence, parents will have chosen a mental health facility and made arrangements for an appointment. When they arrive for this appointment, they will find that the first concern of the professionals at the facility will be to obtain an evaluation of the child's problem. This chapter will describe the types of evaluation that may occur. Based on an evaluation, the staff at the mental health facility will make recommendations concerning treatment. Thus, the evaluation procedure is a critical determinant of the family's later contacts with the facility. It is very important that parents understand and be comfortable with evaluation procedures.

INTERVIEWS

One of the most important evaluation procedures is the interview. In some facilities, these interviews are conducted by a social worker; in other facilities a psychiatrist or a psychologist will conduct the interview. No matter who conducts it, the interview is usually the first interaction between parents and the mental health professionals at the facility. During the interview with the parents, the child may or may not be present. If the child is present, and if parents wish to discuss with the professional an issue that they feel uncomfortable talking about in front of the child, they can indicate this and ask for a private interview. Most mental health professionals will readily provide a parents-only interview when one is requested, although on some occasions some professionals will feel the joint interview to be more valuable and attempt to persuade the parents of this.

In the interview, parents are asked to describe the problem as they see it. They are also asked background questions about themselves and the child; this process is frequently called "taking a history." In some facilities, the emphasis in taking the history is on the child's development; in other facilities, an equal emphasis is on gathering information about the parents' life experiences. Generally speaking, it is important in an evaluation procedure for the mental health professional to have some understanding of both the family's general life style as well as of the specific problem that brought the family to the facility. During the interview, any notes taken by the parent concerning the child's behavior (see pp. 36-38) should be shown to the interviewer. These notes can be extremely helpful in assisting the interviewer to get a clear picture of the child's behavior and of the parents' responses to it prior to coming to the facility.

In some facilities, the child will be interviewed separately from the parents. These separate interviews are undertaken so as to allow children the maximum freedom to discuss their feelings with the mental health professional. If such a separate interview is not offered, but the child wishes to speak to the professional alone, the child or the parents should indicate this to the professional. It is very important in the initial interviews that everyone (child and parents) be able to speak freely with the interviewer. Sometimes important information can be kept from the interviewer because the child doesn't want to say something in front of the parents or the parents in front of the child. Whenever important information is withheld, it will decrease the accuracy and comprehensiveness of the professional's understanding of the family's situation.

INTELLIGENCE TESTING

In dealing with many problems of childhood (for example, mental retardation, learning disabilities, language problems), it is important to have an estimate of the child's general level of intelligence. Thus, one part of many evaluations is to have a psychologist administer an intelligence test to the child. Since "IQ" (intelligence quotient — a measure of intelligence) has become an awesome and frequently fearful object of concern in our society, it may help parents in understanding their child's evaluation to discuss some facts about intelligence tests.

Whenever a child is given an intelligence (IQ) test, the following issues have to be taken into account. Was the IQ test administered properly? An improperly administered test means nothing. Did the examiner establish good rapport with the child? If, for example, a child is intimidated by the examiner and consequently does not behave naturally, all we've learned from the test is what the child will do with certain kinds of materials when in the presence of an intimidating adult. We've learned very little, if anything at all, about what that child can do with these materials under other circumstances.

Test Reliability

Even when the test administration is a good one, there remain issues of reliability and validity. Let us consider reliability first. For a test to mean anything, we must be reasonably confident that the same child given the same test again would obtain the same score. How reliable are IQ tests? In answering this question, it is important to distinguish between the general answer and the specific one. In general, IQ tests are quite reliable; for any specific child, however, any specific test can be unreliable. This problem can be especially worrisome if the child is in an unusual state when the test is administered. If, for example, the child hasn't had enough sleep, or is worried about something, or is thinking about something else other than the materials that are presented, then such a child may obtain an "unreliable" score. That is, when the child is not sleepy, or worried, or distracted, the child may obtain a different score. While no examiner can ever completely discount the possibility that any one test can be unreliable, the examiner can make every effort to make sure that the child is in a proper condition to take the test. The examiner can also advise that the child be reexamined at appropriate intervals so that the unreliability of any one test can be detected.

Test Validity

These issues of test administration and reliability are important ones to consider, but the one issue most important to parents will be the validity of the IQ test. If the test administration was well conducted and the child was in a proper condition to take the test, what does the IQ score mean? What are the implications of that score for the child's future?

First of all, parents need to understand that we cannot really say that intelligence tests measure "intelligence," because psychologists do not yet understand what "intelligence" is. We do know that the intelligence tests that are used in the United States have been shown to measure a variety of intellectual skills that are important if a child is to do well in school in the United States. It is necessary to remember that this relationship is a general one: in general, children who score well on IQ tests also get good grades in school. While this general relationship is well documented, the difficulty comes when a specific child who obtains a specific score and who attends a specific school is considered. Let us look at some of the patterns that can occur.

High IQ score and good performance in school. This pattern confirms the general relationship described above. Parents whose child is described by this pattern have no reason to worry about their child's intellectual functioning.

Low IQ score and poor performance in school. This pattern also confirms the general relationship. Parents whose child is described by this pattern should be concerned about their child's intellectual functioning, but *cannot* conclude that the child is intellectually handicapped. Children who perform poorly both on the IQ test and in school do so because they have not acquired the skills necessary to perform well in both settings. There are a multitude of reasons why this skill acquisition may not have occurred, and a low level of intelligence is only one. Other possible reasons include emotional disturbance, lack of appropriate teaching, and an educationally improverished background. When children show this pattern of behavior, the skilled mental health professional will want to consider all these possibilities. It is important, for example, to find out what the child is doing when out of school. If the child is behaving in intelligent ways in other settings, then low intelligence may not be the problem. Another way to investigate this issue is to provide the child with an intensive educational experience that the mental health professional knows will be individually tailored to the child. If the child makes progress in this situation, then again, low intelligence would not seem to be the problem.

High IQ score and poor performance in school. Assuming the test was properly administered under appropriate conditions, this pattern suggests that something is interfering with the child's learning. What this "something" is can be difficult to clarify; this is the classic pattern of a learning-disabled child, and the difficulty in sorting out what is causing the impairment in learning has been discussed previously (see pp. 21-22; see also pp. 71-73).

Low IQ score and good performance in school. When this pattern occurs, the mental health professional must look at both the test and the school. Sometimes this pattern is an indicator of a poorly administered test; if so, the remedy is quite straightforward: obtain a well-administered test. Sometimes, however, this pattern indicates that the school has standards for good performance that differ from the standards found in most schools. If this is the case, the parents will need to consider their values and the child's welfare most carefully. They may decide to take the IQ score seriously, in which case they would desire the professional to pursue the approaches discussed in the "Low IQ score and poor performance in school" section above. On the other hand, parents may feel that the standards of the school are more important to them than the standards of the dominant society as expressed through the public school system and IQ tests, and may decide to ignore the results of the IQ test. Before making either of these decisions, parents should carefully discuss the situation with the mental health professional. They will want to know what the psychological and educational consequences of either decision might be for their child.

Predictive Validity

Another important issue concerning intelligence tests is their "predictive validity." Professionals ask, and so should parents, "If a young child obtains such-and-such a score on an intelligence test today, how likely is it that (s)he will obtain the same score when (s)he is older?" While a given intelligence test can only measure the child's abilities at the time of testing, it is assumed that this score is similar to that which (s)he would obtain (in the absence of remedial work) as (s)he grows older. No one would care very much about early childhood IQ scores if these scores had no relationship to the IQ scores of the same child when (s)he became older. In order to predict school performance, early childhood IQs must be able to predict the IQ scores that will be obtained for the school-age child.

In approaching this issue, one has to pay attention to differences between different age groups and between different ability groupings. In general, the younger the child the *weaker* the predictive validity of the IQ score. For example, let us consider Amy who is four and Jonathan who is eight. Amy's IQ score will predict the IQ score she will obtain when she is sixteen less well than Jonathan's IQ score will predict his IQ at age sixteen. Also, in general, the poorer the child's performance the *stronger* the predictive validity of the IQ score. A four-year-old child who obtains a *very* poor IQ score is not likely to have more than a poor IQ score as a teenager; a four-year-old child who obtains an average IQ score is unlikely to have a very poor IQ score as an adolescent, but may have an IQ score ranging anywhere from fairly low to very high.

These general observations are of importance for the parent whose child receives an intelligence test. If the child is very young, the parent need not assume that the present IQ will hold for life. If the young child's IQ is, however, quite low, the parent should be aware that the child is unlikely to significantly improve this score and the level of functioning it indicates. Such improvement is not impossible; it is, however, unlikely. As a child becomes older, the parent can have more confidence that the IQ score obtained at those older ages will remain approximately the same throughout the child's development.

Whatever the child's age and whatever the level of functioning indicated by the test, parents should attempt to utilize intelligence test information wisely. First, they probably will not, and probably should not, be told the child's exact IQ score. The reason for withholding the score is that parents (like many educators) can become "hung up" on a number without sufficiently appreciating what that number means. For example, a child may obtain two different IQ scores at two different testings. If parents were given the numbers of these IQ scores, they might conclude, from the scores alone, that the child had gained or lost ground intellectually. Whether, in fact, any real change has occurred will depend on the exact test that was given and the exact scores that were obtained. Parents who are not psychologists do not know enough about intelligence tests and their characteristics to be able to evaluate exact scores. Thus, numbers can be misleading, and in some cases actively harmful. What parents should be told, however, is the general level of functioning (such as "borderline range") indicated by the test and what this means (in this case, that the child is functioning significantly below the average level for his or her age, with some 90% of his or her peers doing better on the test and some 2% doing less well). The second thing parents should be told about a child's performance on an intelligence test is any information that might allow the parents to work with the school in maximizing the child's acquisition of skills. For example, parents might be told that the child is functioning in the average range in skills that do not require communication with others, but in the borderline range for language-related skills. This information lets the parents know that the child has difficulty with language skills, and needs extra help with them. A good teacher can use this information to plan a program for the child.

Finally, parents who are concerned about their child's intellectual functioning will want to have the child retested at appropriate intervals. Usually the mental health professional will suggest this, but if not, the parents can ask about retesting. Retesting is important because it allows parents and professionals to keep track of children's development as they get older, and to see if, as a result of growth or remedial work, they are functioning differently. Retesting is typically done every year or two, and should not be done more than once a year (because the child can learn the test items rather than the skills that the test items are designed to measure).

Special Intelligence Tests

The above discussion refers to children who are capable of taking a "regular" intelligence test—who can adequately speak, see, and coordinate the movements of their limbs. For children who have special difficulties (such as deafness, blindness, communication problems, paralysis), special tests have to be utilized. In this special testing, it is particularly important to give the child the test that will assess his or her optimal ability. We already know that such children are handicapped; what we want to know is how well they can do when we give them a test with which their handicap doesn't interfere. Parents whose child has a specific handicap should be sure that their child receives a test that has been designed for just such children.

ABILITY TESTS

In addition to testing more general intellectual functions, there is frequently the need to test the child's skills on specific, usually academic, subjects. One widely used test for this purpose examines the grade level of a child's skills in reading, spelling, and arithmetic. In addition, there are numerous tests for examining a child's reading in terms not only of grade level but of approaches to reading and lower-level skills underlying the reading process. All ability testing should be done in conjunction with consultation with the school. The child who performs well in the mental health facility but is failing in school is a very different child from one who performs poorly both in the facility and in school.

PROJECTIVE TESTS

Projective tests are tests designed to assess a person's personality. It was once thought that showing people pictures and/or inkblots and recording their spontaneous responses to such materials would reveal what really concerned and motivated them. Since the pictures and inkblots are somewhat ambiguous and vague, it was believed that people would describe them in ways that reflected their personality. This hypothesis—stating that people would "project" their inner psychology onto ambiguous external objects—is called the "projective hypothesis."

In recent years, there has been much criticism of projective tests. The projective hypothesis is not well proven, and many of the tests themselves have not stood up well to scientific investigation. Some psychologists, however, continue to utilize them, and some psychiatrists continue to ask psychologists to use them. Criticism of projective testing is particularly pertinent with young children of preschool or elementary school age. Many projective tests were designed to be used with adults, and the usefulness of such adult tests with children is highly debatable.

Rather than becoming enmeshed in a still ongoing professional controversy, parents can consider adopting the following attitude toward projective tests. If the mental health facility wishes to use projective tests with a child, this use is not in itself harmful. Indeed, many psychologists use projective tests not as "tests," but as additional interview material. Sometimes young children have difficulty in talking about their feelings; in these cases, more indirect approaches, such as having them tell a story about a picture, can help them talk more freely. Furthermore, even when used as tests and even with young children, projective tests will be most useful and most accurate when they are used in conjunction with other information about the child and family that is gathered in other ways (such as interviews, inventories, and observation).

If parents become concerned that an inadequate or inappropriate evaluation is being conducted with their child, they should inquire about the use of projective tests. They can ask:

1. Is the identification of my child's problem being made solely on the basis of a projective test?
2. If other information is being considered, what is this other information?
3. If other information is not being considered, why isn't it?
4. How important were the projective test results in the understanding of my child's problem?

If the answer to the first question is yes and the answer to the third question is unsatisfactory, the parent might be well advised to obtain a second opinion from another mental health professional or facility (see Chapter 7). Specification of a child's problem should not be based *solely* on projective tests. Alternatively, even with a no to the first question, the parent may feel that the answers to questions 2 and 4 indicate too much reliance on projective tests and too little consideration of other information, and might in this case also desire a second opinion. If, on the other hand, projective tests are just one part of a more comprehensive evaluation with other information being utilized, and/or the projective tests are used more as interview materials than as "tests," then the parent can probably assume that the facility is making an appropriate use of projective tests.

INVENTORIES

Some tests are designed to assess an individual's pattern of behavior. When children are being evaluated, these tests usually consist of *inventories* of the child's behavior. That is, either the child or someone (parent, teacher) familiar with the child will be asked whether the child does a certain behavior, and/or how much (s)he does it, and/or how strongly (s)he does it. Many behaviors are typically asked about in an inventory. The answers received are then analyzed according to specific instructions for an individual inventory and usually yield some score (or scores) indicating whether the child is within the normal range for specific types of behavior.[1]

---

[1] There is another type of psychological test that is neither a projective test nor an inventory. These tests usually give a number of statements (for example, "I love my mother," "I worry a lot"), and respondents are asked to agree or disagree with each of these statements. The respondent's pattern of answers is used to indicate whether or not the respondent is similar to various groups of people who have been identified as having certain specified psychological problems. Because this type of test requires the person being evaluated to read and respond to the items, it is used less with children than are inventories, which typically allow an adult to respond to the test items if necessary or desirable.

Inventories are not without their problems. One major factor of concern is the standardization group that was used as the basis for creating the test. For instance, if the standardization group consisted only of children of professors, then children of people who are not professors may appear abnormal when compared to this standardization group. In reality, however, the children of people who are not professors may be quite normal (and, perhaps, compared to the general population, the children of professors may be the ones who are unusual). Thus it is important that only inventories be used that have adequate standardization groups (that is, groups that are representative of the entire population).

Apart from this problem (which can be hard for a layperson to evaluate), inventories may be considered to be somewhat similar to projective tests. They should not be the sole basis for an evaluation and other information should be utilized. Inventories can also be used as interview materials rather than as "tests." The professional may find it helpful to ask parents (or teachers or the child) to answer the questions on the inventory, not so much so that a score can be obtained, but so that an orderly, systematic picture of what behaviors the child engages in, under what circumstances, can be elicited.

OBSERVATION

One of the most valuable assessment techniques available to the mental health professional is observation. Indeed, in an ideal world, assessment of a child's problem would be based on 24-hour observation of that child. Through such continual observation, we would know exactly what the child does, when and how (s)he does it, when it causes problems, and when it is beneficial. Unfortunately, we do not live in such an ideal world; we live in a real one in which 24-hour observation of one child by professional observers is not usually possible. We are able, however, to observe *samples* of a child's life. The systematic and detailed observation of these samples constitutes an important and increasingly utilized approach to assessment.

Observations at the Facility

Some observations may be made at the mental health facility. The parent may be asked to work or play with the child while the mental health professional observes. Another approach is for the mental health professional to get another professional to observe the professional's interview of the family. Many important patterns of family interaction can be found through these types of observation.

Observations at Home

Observations of the family at the facility suffer from the fact that parental and child behavior at the facility may not be typical behavior. The facility can seem a strange and sometimes frightening place and may promote behavior that is unusual and only occurs in strange and frightening places. One remedy for this problem is to observe the family at home. At first, the family will feel awkward and uncomfortable in the presence of an observer. For most families and with most observers, however, this initial discomfort soon fades away and the family engages in its typical routine. Observations of the family at home provide excellent information about the child's behavior and the parents' response to this behavior.

Observations at School

Many childhood problems are, at least in part, school problems. If school problems are reported, it is very important that the professional assess these problems by observing the child at school. Mental health professionals are able to conduct such observations without making the child feel uncomfortable or unduly self-conscious.

In summary, then, parents who are asked for their permission to be observed should feel positively about this request. The professional who wishes to observe want to do so to ensure the best and most accurate assessment of the child's problem. Indeed, if parents are having a difficult time describing certain features of the child's behavior, they might ask that the professional come to observe the family and "see for him/herself."

OTHER TYPES OF EVALUATION PROCESSES

Sometimes other types of evaluation processes are important in the assessment of the child. Thus, not infrequently (see Chapter 2), physical examinations of the child are necessary to see whether any physical problem is involved. Neurological examinations are sometimes recommended if the child behaves in ways that suggest that the nervous system may be impaired. If the child appears to have a communication problem, an examination by a speech and language specialist will be recommended. If the child has difficulties in motor coordination, an evaluation by a physical therapist may be recommended. And so forth. There are many, many possible additional evaluation processes that may be recommended, depending on the child's problem. In each case, the goal is to obtain the most complete picture possible of the child's behavior and to consider all the possible characteristics of the child that may be involved.

EXAMPLES OF POSSIBLE EVALUATIONS

In order to make the above discussion of evaluation techniques more meaningful to the parent, the following examples of possible evaluations are offered. These examples are not meant to indicate the perfect evaluation for the specific problem. Rather, they are presented as examples of what type of evaluation might be conducted for a specific problem. Thus, the examples are meant as general guidelines and not as prescribed procedures. Parents whose child has one of the following problems and who are offered a different type of evaluation procedure should discuss these differences with the professional with whom they are working. In the majority of cases, the professional will then be able to show how his or her evaluation is more suitable for the individual child being evaluated. If, however, parents do not find the proposed evaluation suitable, they should consider consulting another mental health professional or facility. (See Chapter 7 for discussion of obtaining second opinions.)

MENTAL RETARDATION

Let us consider the Warrens who bring their four-year-old daughter Joan to a mental health facility for evaluation. The Warrens indicate that they are concerned that Joan is mentally retarded.

EVALUATION

- Interview with Warrens—Joan may be present at the interview.
- Intelligence testing with Joan—in many facilities, the parents may observe this testing.

- Observation of Joan in the home and in her preschool.
- Possible supplementary evaluations: speech and language; physical examination with neurological screening; physical therapist.

From these evaluation procedures, the following information will be gathered: a complete developmental history of Joan from birth to present; Joan's current level of intellectual functioning; Joan's current level of behavior within the family and with peers; Joan's level of language and motor functioning; and Joan's physical status. This information will help to answer the following questions:

- Is Joan currently functioning within the mentally retarded range?
- How do her language and motor development relate to her overall intellectual functioning?
- How does her social behavior relate to her level of overall intellectual functioning?
- Were there prenatal or birth problems that might lead to mental retardation?

In answering these questions, the professional can decide whether or not Joan is mentally retarded. The professional can also begin to draw a picture of Joan as an individual, with individual strengths and weaknesses. This picture will be useful in helping the parents anticipate what sort of progress to expect from Joan in the future and in assisting with educational programs to maximize this progress.

Learning Disabilities

In evaluating a child for learning disabilities, several factors must be taken into account. First, there is the comparison between the child's overall intellectual skills and his or her achievements in specific learning tasks. Only children who show overall cognitive skills that are at least average for their age but have less-than-average achievement are considered learning-disabled (see pp. 21-22). Second, the entire complex issue of cause and effect must be addressed. If a child is learning more poorly than would be expected from his or her general overall intellectual functioning, what accounts for this? It could be that (s)he learns differently from other children, in which case an effort must be made to find a more helpful teaching approach. It could be that his or her learning difficulties stem from emotional difficulties (s)he is having at home or in school, and thus need to be treated.

Or it could be that (s)he has an unusually poor teacher and no one is learning very much from this teacher, in which case changing teachers should be considered. While the assessment procedures themselves may not be able to answer this second issue definitively, the assessment should provide at least some good possibilities.

For an example of how the possibility of a learning disability might be evaluated, let us consider the Matthews who bring their eight-year-old son Bryan to a mental health facility.

EVALUATION

Interview with parents	To obtain history of Bryan's learning problem. To find out if his parents had similar problems in school.
Interview with child	To find out Bryan's ideas about whether he has a learning problem, and if so, what causes it.
Interview with teacher	To find out his or her ideas about whether Bryan has a learning problem, and if so, what causes it.
Individually administered intelligence test	To find out Bryan's general overall intellectual skills.
Individually administered achievement test	To find out level of Bryan's achievement in specific learning areas.
Individually administered special tests such as reading tests, tests for auditory and visual discrimination	To find out if Bryan has a specific disability that may underlie his learning problem. The reading test can also help pinpoint Bryan's specific difficulty in reading (if this is at least a part of his learning problem) and generate ideas for remedial teaching.
Evaluations by an audiometrist and ophthalmologist	To rule out possible hearing and visual difficulties that might produce a learning problem.
Observation of Bryan at school	To assess how Bryan functions in the classroom.
Observation of Bryan at home	To assess how Bryan functions at home.

These procedures should help to answer the following questions:

1. Does Bryan have a learning disability?
2. If so, what is the specific nature of that disability? (For example: all school skills below average; or only reading below average with good comprehension but slow speed.)
3. What are the most likely causes of the difficulty? [For example: (a) specific

learning disability without other problems; (b) social and emotional problems that seem to underlie the learning problem; or (c) social and emotional problems that seem to be caused by the learning problem.]

These findings can point to possible treatment approaches. For example, if (a) were the case, treatment would probably center on improving Bryan's learning skills. If (b) were the case, treatment might first try to help Bryan emotionally, with remedial learning programs becoming gradually more important. If (c) were the case, the treatment might focus equally on Bryan's learning and Bryan's social and emotional difficulties.

Behavior Problem

When parents bring a child to a mental health facility with what they consider a behavior problem, the assessment should be directed toward two issues: Is there a behavior problem? And, if so, what can help to change it? These questions may best be answered by obtaining a careful record of the child's behavior and of the reactions by other people to that behavior. In this example of evaluation procedures, let us consider the Baker family. This is a single-parent family. Mrs. Baker, recently divorced, brings her eleven-year-old son Kevin to the mental health facility. She is concerned that Kevin is too aggressive.

EVALUATION

Interview with parent	To get her history and description of the problem. Notes taken by Mrs. Baker (see pp. 36-38) can be especially helpful.
Interview with Kevin	To get his view of whether he has a problem and, if so, what could help him with it.
Interview with Kevin's teacher(s)	To get their view of whether he has a problem and, if so, what could help him with it.
Observation of Kevin at home	To obtain a careful record of Kevin's behavior and other people's responses to it.
Observation of Kevin at school	To obtain a careful record of Kevin's behavior and other people's responses to it.
Additional possible sources of information	Evaluations of intellectual functioning, academic achievement, physical condition, and language skills.

These procedures should enable the professional to decide whether Kevin has a behavior problem, or whether Mrs. Baker has unrealistic expectations about the child's behavior. Either state of affairs may warrant some professional help. In the former case, the program would center around trying to help Kevin reduce his aggression and find other, more appropriate behaviors that satisfy his needs; in the latter case, the professional could help Mrs. Baker work out more realistic expectations for her child.

It is hoped that these examples of possible evaluations will help parents know what to expect when they initially take their child to a mental health facility. Different evaluations will be given by different facilities to different children with different problems. All evaluations should share, however, the goals of deciding whether there is a problem and, if so, specifying the factors that could affect it and that should therefore be addressed in treatment.

> "What is it you want to buy?" the Sheep said at last,
> looking up for a moment from her knitting. "I don't *quite*
> know yet," Alice said very gently. "I should like to look all
> round me first, if I might."
>
> *Through the Looking-Glass*

What Kinds of Treatment May a Mental Health Facility Recommend for My Child?

CHAPTER 6

The purposes of the evaluation procedures described in the previous chapter are to decide whether treatment is necessary and, if so, to determine what kind of treatment should be recommended. While in some instances the evaluation itself may be very time-consuming and require great effort from both the professional staff and the family, neither professionals nor family members should lose sight of these eventual goals of the evaluation.

Once the evaluation is completed, the mental health professional will meet with the parents and child (either separately or together) to discuss the results of the evaluation and to make recommendations about treatment. Parents need to listen very carefully to the treatment recommendations and make sure they understand exactly what is being recommended; only then are they in a position to evaluate the treatment recommendation and decide whether or not to accept it.

This chapter will give a brief description of a variety of types of treatment that might be recommended by mental health professionals. Its aim is to make it easier for the parent to understand any specific treatment recommendation. Having read this chapter, a parent can receive a specific treatment recommendation *in context:* The parent will be aware of what other types of treatment exist, but that are *not* being recommended. The parent should then be prepared to evaluate the treatment recommendation; Chapter 7 offers suggestions about how a parent can go about doing this.

In order to facilitate your reading of this chapter as well as Chapter 7, Table 6-1 provides a guide to the pages in each chapter where each type of treatment is discussed. It is suggested that the reader go through each chapter in its entirety so that the context of both chapters becomes clear. With this background in hand, Table 6-1 can then assist you in examining any particular type(s) of treatment in more detail.

NO TREATMENT

A recommendation for no treatment is probably a fairly infrequent recommendation, but it can be given. When such a recommendation is made, it indicates to parents that the mental health professionals who conducted the evaluation believe that no further contact with mental health professionals is necessary for the family. This recommendation would be made when the professionals conclude that the child's behavior is within the range of behaviors displayed by children without mental health problems and that the parents' behavior and expectations are basically realistic and reasonable.

MODIFICATION OF PARENTAL EXPECTATIONS

The evaluation may indicate to the mental health professional that the child's behavior is reasonably normal and healthy, but that parental expectations are unrealistic. In this case, the professional may recommend that the parents discuss their expectations with a mental health professional so as to gain a more realistic picture of what to expect from their child. This form of treatment should be relatively short-term (perhaps eight to ten sessions). The goal of this treatment is specific change in parental expectations about the child.

TABLE 6-1
A Guide to Specific Types of Mental Health Treatments.
Discussed in Chapters 6 and 7.

Treatment Type	Chapter 6 Page Number(s)	Chapter 7 Page Number(s)
No treatment	76	96
Modification of parental expectations	76	96-99
Psychotherapy	78-82	99-105
Individual	80-81	100-101
Play	81	*
Couples	81	*
Family	82	101-102
Group	82	101
Behavior therapy	82-85	105-110
Reinforcement	83	*
Time-out	83	*
Desensitization	84-85	*
Child-rearing counseling	85	110
Parent effectiveness training (PET)	85	110
Supportive therapy	85	110-111
Education	85-87	111-113
Medication	87-88	113-119
Inpatient treatment	88-90	119-130
Psychological treatments	89	126-127
Physical treatments	89-90	127-130
Medication	89-90	127
Electroconvulsive therapy	90	127-129
Psychosurgery	90	129-130
Supplementary treatments	90-91	130-131

*Not discussed.

PSYCHOTHERAPY

Psychotherapy is a term that can be used in a variety of ways. Sometimes it is used in general sense to indicate any kind of nonphysical treatment of psychological problems; in this sense, any treatment described in this chapter that does not use medication, electroshock, or surgery can be considered "psychotherapy." Frequently, however, psychotherapy is used in a more specific sense. In this case, it designates those types of psychological treatment in which the major activity that occurs is that the therapist and the client[1] talk with each other, *and* in which the goal of the therapy is personality change. The latter characteristic is quite important. Later in this chapter, a form of treatment called "behavior therapy" will be described. In behavior therapy, the major activity also consists of therapist and client talking with each other. The aim of behavior therapy, however, is typically for change in more specific behaviors rather than change in that sum total of a person's feelings, beliefs, thoughts, and behavior that can be called "personality."

In addition to distinguishing between psychotherapy and behavior therapy, it is necessary to distinguish among different types of psychotherapy. While all psychotherapists share the emphasis on changing the client's personality, there are many other aspects of therapy on which they differ. These differences arise because different psychotherapists follow different theories about how psychological problems come about and about how to help the client work with these problems. One way to introduce parents to these differences is to describe three general types of theoretical orientation that have influenced many psychotherapists. This description is by no means an exhaustive one; only major theoretical orientations are described. For a more inclusive and much more detailed discussion of theories of psychotherapy, the reader would be well advised to consult a book on theories of therapy such as *Theory and Practice of Counseling and Psychotherapy* by Gerald Corey (Monterey, Calif.: Brooks/Cole, 1977).

Theories of Psychotherapy

PSYCHOANALYSIS

Psychoanalysis is based primarily on the personality theory of Sigmund Freud (1856-1939). Freud's theory states that psychological problems in

---

[1]Some mental health professionals call the people for whom they provide services "patients"; others call them "clients." I personally prefer the term "client" and will use this term throughout the discussion of both psychotherapy and behavior therapy.

both children and adults arise from unconscious conflicts within the person. Typically, these conflicts result from the collision of instinctual impulses (particularly sexual ones) with prohibitions against the expression of these impulses.

In psychoanalysis, an effort is made to uncover the unconscious conflict, bring it to the client's awareness, and help the client deal more realistically with it. Psychoanalysis was originally applied almost exclusively to adults. Through the work of several analysts such as Anna Freud (Freud's daughter) and Melanie Klein, practitioners began to apply analysis to children. Many child guidance clinics are characterized by a strong emphasis on psychoanalytic principles.

In classic psychoanalysis (also called orthodox psychoanalysis), the child is treated individually. While other members of the family may also be seen in their own separate analyses, no effort is made in the typical case to treat the family as a unit. It is believed that by helping children work through their conflicts (either through talking or playing with the child) and helping them come to recognize these conflicts, children will understand themselves better and be able to make more realistic choices about what they want and what they want to do. Typically, only "neurotic" children are offered psychoanalysis. In practice, this means that white, middle- to upper-socioeconomic-class, intelligent, talkative children who are more inhibited than aggressive are most frequently offered psychoanalysis.

INTERPERSONAL THERAPY

The major figure associated with interpersonal therapy is Harry Stack Sullivan (1892-1949), although other well-known psychotherapists (for example, Karen Horney, 1885-1952) have also emphasized interpersonal factors in the development of psychological problems. Therapists adopting an interpersonal orientation believe that psychological problems arise from difficulties in interpersonal relationships. They stress the need for interpersonal security in order for the person to develop normally.

Interpersonal therapists are likely to use a variety of treatment approaches. Because of their interpersonal orientation, such therapists often work with groups of individuals (children's groups, parents' groups, or family groups). They may also utilize individual psychotherapy, either by itself or in combination with group treatment. Their typical emphasis in therapy is that people need to understand their relations with others and need to learn how to go about establishing satisfying relationships. With children, a typical emphasis would be on creating better communication and more trust between parents and child.

CLIENT-CENTERED THERAPY

The founder of client-centered therapy is Carl Rogers (b. 1902). Client-centered therapy is based on the assumption that the reason a person has psychological difficulties is that the person is not being himself or herself and is acting unnaturally because of external pressures. The client-centered approach seeks to help a person "self-actualize," to become fully his or her own person. A client-centered—or, to use a term that more recently has come to be applied to this orientation, humanistic—therapist might well see a child in individual play therapy. Play therapy would serve to emphasize to the child the therapist's respect for the child's free and creative expression.

Forms of Psychotherapy

As indicated in the above description of theories of psychotherapy, different therapists may emphasize different forms of therapy—such as individual, family, or play. The following outline briefly describes these different forms of therapy.

INDIVIDUAL THERAPY

Individual psychotherapy may be recommended for the child and/or for one or both parents. In individual therapy, the person meets on a regular schedule with the therapist. What is discussed between therapist and client will vary depending on the therapist's theoretical orientation and the client's difficulties. Some theories of therapy recommend basic procedures for all therapists to follow with all clients. Other theories are less specific about procedures so that therapists can follow different procedures with different clients. In addition, some therapists consider themselves "eclectic" in orientation—that is, willing to apply several different theories of therapy to their understanding of human behavior. Eclectic therapists typically utilize a number of different procedures and try to tailor their procedures to the specific client. Two of the more structured approaches to psychotherapy will be described below. These two types of approaches provide an indication of the range of therapist behavior and duration of therapy that can currently be found among psychotherapists.

Psychoanalysis requires a certain set of procedures to be followed in individual psychotherapy. The basic structure of psychoanalysis is the same for every client: the client is instructed to tell the analyst everything that comes to mind during therapy (this is called "free association") and, from time to time, the analyst will "interpret" the psychological meaning of the client's statements. Analytic sessions are typically held for one hour three to five days a week, and a full analysis takes a very long time, with two to three years being considered fairly short and six years or more not being uncommon.

Client-centered (or Rogerian) therapy also has an unvarying basic format. The client-centered therapist will not tell the client what to do, but will be "nondirective" and support the client's initiatives in therapy. Also, client-centered therapists will not interpret their clients' statements, but will try to assist their clients to hear themselves more clearly and to obtain a clearer perspective on their own thoughts and feelings. Client-centered therapy is usually conducted in one or two sessions each week and, compared to psychoanalysis, lasts a shorter time, with several months to a year being fairly common.

PLAY THERAPY

This is a form of individual psychotherapy sometimes recommended for young children. In play therapy, the guiding principle is that the child will express his or her feelings through play rather than through conversation. Exact procedures and duration of therapy will vary greatly depending on the therapist's orientation and the child's difficulties.

COUPLES THERAPY

This is a form of individual psychotherapy in which both parents meet with a therapist. Typically, the goal of couples therapy is to improve the psychological functioning of each member of the pair. Sometimes this will strengthen the existing relationship between the couple, but at other times individual improvement appears to be possible only outside the relationship. Thus, there is no necessary commitment on the part of the therapist or by the parental couple to maintaining the marriage. This type of therapy should be distinguished from child-rearing counseling described later in this chapter. In couples therapy, the child's problems are addressed only as one of any number of difficulties that the couple may experience together or singly, whereas in child-rearing counseling the child's behavior and parents' response to it constitute the major focus of the interaction between professional and client. Exact procedures and duration of couples therapy will vary greatly depending on the therapist's theoretical orientation and the couple's difficulties.

FAMILY THERAPY

The evaluation may indicate that at least one significant problem area concerns communication among family members. The professional may then recommend family therapy. In family therapy, all family members come together with a mental health professional and discuss their relationships with one another. Procedures and duration of family therapy will depend on the family, its difficulties, and the therapist's theoretical orientation.

GROUP THERAPY

Group therapy consists of several people, usually around four to eight, meeting with one or more therapists (usually one, sometimes two). A typical goal in group therapy is to improve each person's skills in relating to others. It is believed helpful to have the person actually relate to others in the presence of the therapist so that the therapist can assist the person in becoming aware of his or her problems in interpersonal relationships. In the treatment of childhood problems, a group may be recommended for the child (usually with peers) and/or for the parents. If a group is recommended for the parents, they may be urged to go to a group together or separately. If they go separately, typically the focus of the group would be on each of them as individuals rather than as parents. If they go together, the group may focus on them as individuals or may be more child-oriented and focus on their relationship with their child. Procedures and duration of group therapy are highly variable and depend on the therapist's orientation, the group members, and the focus of the group.

BEHAVIOR THERAPY

Behavior therapy is a relatively new approach to psychological problems. Its emphasis is on behavior change. Behavior therapy tends to address problems more specifically than psychotherapy, is less concerned with finding out the original cause of the problem, and usually takes less time. Behavior therapy may be conducted by the therapist seeing the parents (alone or together), or the child, or the entire family. It is quite common for a behavior therapist to want to talk with different family members at different times during therapy. Behavior therapists also conduct groups for parents and/or children. There are many different types of behavior therapy. Described below are some of the ones most frequently used with children.

Reinforcement Management

Reinforcement management programs are conducted under the assumption that behaviors that are reinforced (rewarded) will increase, while behaviors that are not rewarded will decrease. A behavior therapist may, for example, find from observing a certain child that this child receives attention when he misbehaves and is ignored when he behaves. This situation amounts to rewarding the child with attention when he behaves in an undesirable way, and not rewarding him when he behaves in a desirable way. This, of course, would be the exact opposite of that which most of us would want for the child. Thus, a reinforcement management program might teach the parents to observe the child's "good" behavior and to reward it consistently. The parents might also be instructed to ignore the "bad" behaviors. This kind of approach can be utilized with many different behaviors both at home and at school.

Time-Out

Time-out is a variation of the reinforcement management program described above. Sometimes it is found that rewarding an individual child for "good" behavior and ignoring "bad" behavior is not sufficient; the child continues to engage in many more "bad" than "good" behaviors. Sometimes time-out is recommended to help with this. Time-out consists of placing the child in a boring environment immediately after he or she misbehaves. If the time-out takes place in the child's room, it is frequently necessary to take out toys and other entertainment items so that the room is boring and uninteresting to the child. After a specified time period, usually quite short (such as two minutes), the child is allowed out of his or her room. It is critical when using time-out to reward the child consistently for good behavior. By combining rewards for the desired behavior and time-out for undesirable behavior, it is believed that the child will learn to associate being placed in a dull environment with misbehaving and being rewarded with behaving appropriately. Being rewarded is obviously preferable to having "time-out," and for many children this will result in increasing the desired behavior.

A Word to the Wise. Reinforcement management and time-out procedures should sound very familiar to most parents. Rewarding "good" behavior and responding to "bad" behavior by telling the child, "Go to your room" are certainly not ideas original to behavior therapy. Most parents and teachers have followed these principles without ever hearing of behavior therapy. Parents should be aware, however, that behavior therapy may not be so simple. Many abuses can result if these principles are applied to a child by an untrained person. Time-out can be interpreted to mean punishing children by sticking them in a closet for hours at a time. The wrong target behavior can be addressed such that children are rewarded for behaviors that will not actually help them or are not rewarded at all because they are unable to perform the behavior the parents desire. All of these approaches represent a misunderstanding of behavior therapy and can harm the child.

Thus, in general, parents should approach behavior therapy just as they would approach psychotherapy. For a child with psychological problems, these behavioral techniques are therapies that should be conducted or supervised only by qualified professionals. If the parent would like a fuller discussion of these principles—either for better understanding of a behavior therapy that is being recommended or for considering how these principles can operate in everyday family life—there are books available written specifically for the lay public. One that I would highly recommend is *Families: Applications of Social Learning to Family Life* by G.R. Patterson (Champaign, Ill.: Research Press, 1971).

Desensitization

Desensitization is another form of behavior therapy. Desensitization would be used with a child who has excessive fears. It is believed that these fears can be reduced by gradually exposing the child to aspects of the feared object that do not evoke fear. Thus, for example, with a child who feared school, a desensitization program might take the child step by step, nearer and nearer the school, always making sure the child is relaxed and unafraid before going closer. This procedure may also sound familiar to parents, since many parents believe in introducing children gradually to things that are new or that might frighten them. Proper use of desensitization in treatment, however, is also a professional activity. The technique could be abused—for example, by taking the child too close to the feared object, or by making a mistake about what the child feared (for example, thinking the child fears school when the child actually fears other children). It is strongly urged that parents not try to attempt desensitization on their own when a strong fear is involved, but always consult a professional on this.

CHILD-REARING COUNSELING

In child-rearing counseling, the parents receive advice on how best to cope with their child. The goal of such counseling is improved parent-child relations and improved child behavior. The duration of such counseling is seldom very long. It would be unusual, for example, for child-rearing counseling to last longer than one year.

Parent Effectiveness Training (PET)

Parent effectiveness training (PET) is a structured form of child-rearing counseling in which parents attend classes with other parents where techniques for more effective parenting are taught. Typically, these classes are for parents whose children are not experiencing any mental health problems. However, in their emphasis on how to improve everyday parenting activities, PET classes may be helpful to parents whose children do have mental health problems, particularly when these problems are not severe, PET classes would not be recommended as the primary type of treatment for parents whose child has severe psychological difficulties.

SUPPORTIVE THERAPY

Supportive therapy seeks to help the family or individual members maintain their optimum psychological functioning. It is more a maintenance procedure than a change procedure. The length of supportive therapy varies greatly, usually in proportion to the client's need for support.

EDUCATION

Parents may not usually think of education as a kind of treatment for psychological problems. And yet for children, being educated can be one of the most important experiences that will determine their future. Thus, no psychological treatment for children can ignore their educational experiences.

Another misconception that many parents (and others) share is the notion that "special education" classes are a "dumping ground" for the intellectually retarded. Modern educators are trying hard to create a more positive view and to improve the actual education that goes on in special education classes. The nature of special education is of particular concern for parents whose child has psychological or intellectual problems that interfere with his or her learning.

As indicated in Chapter 5, evaluation of a child's school performance (*school* being broadly defined to include nurseries and preschools as well as later school grades) is an important aspect of any general evaluation of a child. If it is determined that the child is having difficulties — academic, social, or both — in school, then treatment approaches designed to improve the child's performance in school will be recommended.

These recommendations can cover a wide range. For some children, it will be suggested that they continue in a "regular" school with a "regular" program but change teachers or schools. For some children, however, something in addition to a "regular" program at a "regular" school will be recommended. I suggest that parents regard any such additions as *special education*. I also urge parents to try to convice their communities and school boards to take this broad view of special education and to make a commitment to providing whatever type of special education is needed to whatever child needs it. (See Chapter 10 for further discussion of parents' activities in improving educational resources for children with psychological problems.)

There are many different types of special education that can be recommended. Some of the easiest types to obtain are supplements to the child's regular school program; for example, some children might benefit from having extra classes in reading or a tutor in math. More elaborate programs might require that children spend some part of their school day in a special classroom that is designed to help them with their problems; these classrooms can be found in some school districts for children with behavioral problems (usually those who are excessively aggressive or hyperactive), for children with language problems, and/or for children with learning disabilities. These classrooms are staffed by specially trained teachers and supervised aides, all of whom work to help these children with their specific problems and then return them for the rest of the day to their regular classrooms.

Sometimes it is not sufficient to have a child in a special classroom for only part of a day; it may be necessary to have him or her in such a classroom all day. Again, such classrooms may be designed to handle one or more of many types of problems: behavior problems, language problems, learning disabilities, mental retardation. Some of these classrooms will seek to place the child back in a regular classroom at the end of a specified period of time or when the child is judged to be ready for a regular classroom. Some of these classrooms, especially those for the mentally retarded, will not seek to place the child in a regular classroom, but instead will work to maximize the child's learning in a sequence of learning experiences specially designed to benefit children with this difficulty.

As there are special classrooms, so there are special schools for the emotionally disturbed and for the mentally retarded. Some of these schools are outpatient facilities; the child lives at home while attending class at the school. Some of them are inpatient facilities; the child lives at the school. Depending on the school and the individual child, sometimes the goal will be to return the child to a regular school, while sometimes the goal will be to complete the child's education at the school.

MEDICATION

Medication for children with psychological problems is less frequently prescribed than medication for adults with such problems. One reason for this is that fewer medicines have been found to be helpful for children than have been found to be helpful for adults. Another reason is that administering medication to a child is always more dangerous than to an adult. Children are growing, developing organisms, and a medication that would not harm an adult can have damaging effects on a child.

This book will make no effort to describe the many types of medication that could be prescribed for children. Probably the most important issue for parents who are told to give a particular medication to their child is their evaluation of this medication and its effects. Ways to evaluate medication are discussed in Chapter 7.

One increasingly common instance when medication is prescribed will, however, be mentioned. Many parents are probably familiar with the recent practice of prescribing medication to treat hyperactivity. The medication most frequently prescribed is methylphenidate (trade name: Ritalin). For most people, Ritalin acts as an energizer, an "upper," but with some hyperactive children it has been found to act as a "downer" and to calm them. Ritalin is prescribed to help the child pay attention better and be less easily distracted, thus learning more effectively in school. Parental evaluation of treatment of hyperactivity by Ritalin is extremely important; parents with a hyperactive child should be sure to read the discussion of this kind of evaluation provided in Chapter 7.

INPATIENT TREATMENT

The approaches to children's psychological problems noted above are given to children and families who continue to live together. These are called "outpatient" treatments in that the child remains with his or her family and comes to the clinic or special school for periodic visits. There are also, however, treatments that can be delivered in an "inpatient" setting, where the child lives most of the time at a hospital or school, although he or she may go home for visits. This section discusses the various treatment approaches that might be used in an inpatient setting.

In discussing inpatient treatment, the first issue involves the recommendation for the child to live away from home. There can be many different reasons for such a recommendation, for example:

1. The child needs intensive care that cannot be provided for a child living at home.
2. Under ideal circumstances, outpatient care could be provided, but the family situation is too overburdened or too stressful to make this practical.
3. The family wishes to have the child live away from home, either temporarily or permanently.
4. The family setting is actively harmful to the child.

In recent years, the first reason noted above has become less and less significant. Most forms of treatment for children are available to them on an outpatient basis. In some instances, however, this requires tremendous cooperation, energy, and strong motivation from the parents. To say that outpatient treatment is theoretically possible doesn't mean that it is practically feasible for every child in every family.

When a recommendation is made for the child to live away from home, parents must evaluate this recommendation very carefully. This evaluation process will be discussed in Chapter 7. In order to evaluate a recommendation for inpatient care, parents should make sure they understand the goals of the suggested treatment. Goals may range from relatively short periods of inpatient care (to give the other family members some rest from coping with a difficult child, or to provide a special "push" to attempt to obtain some improvement in the child's behavior) to anticipated lifelong institutionalization.

Psychological Treatments Available in Inpatient Facilities

All of the treatments noted for children living at home may be offered to children living in a group home, hospital, or school. They may receive individual psychotherapy, group therapy, behavior therapy, and/or special education. Their parents may participate — either at the facility or in their local community in supportive, group, child-rearing, or behavior therapy. One treatment available in inpatient facilities that is not available for children living at home is "milieu therapy" for the child. While this term has often been misused, sometimes only meaning any kind of custodial care, its original meaning referred to a distinct kind of therapy. The notion was that a child's problem might be so extensive or intensive or long-lasting that periodic treatment would be insufficient. It was believed that the child needed therapeutic attention every moment of every day throughout the child's environment. Thus, in a facility that utilizes true milieu therapy, every moment in the child's day is utilized as part of the child's treatment.

Physical Treatments Available in Inpatient Facilities

The following types of physical treatments of psychological problems may only be administered under the supervision of a physician (M.D.). Medication may be administered in any kind of inpatient facility, although its use is most prevalent in psychiatric wards or hospitals. ECT and psychosurgery (see below) would not be offered in a group home or in a school specializing in mental health care for children. ECT and psychosurgery might be offered by some psychiatric departments or hospitals.

MEDICATION
In general, children who have the most severe problems (such as psychosis or severe mental retardation) tend to be more often hospitalized than children with milder problems. Thus, it is not surprising that children

in hospitals are more likely to receive medication than children outside of hospitals. Again, this is a treatment that parents have to evaluate most carefully (see Chapter 7).

ELECTROCONVULSIVE THERAPY (ECT).

In electroconvulsive therapy, the person is administered electric shocks that are strong enough to cause a convulsion, but not strong enough to be a threat to life. The person is asleep when the shock is administered and is not aware of the convulsion. This treatment is utilized more with adults than with children, but has sometimes been utilized with children. In order to administer ECT to a child, the hospital must have a signed consent form from the parent. Before agreeing to sign such a form, parents will want to carefully evaluate this treatment (see Chapter 7).

PSYCHOSURGERY

Psychosurgery refers to operations on the brain that attempt to affect behavior. The best known of these procedures is the lobotomy. Again, this treatment is utilized more with adults than with children, but some psychosurgical procedures have been utilized with adolescents. Parents must give their consent for such an operation and, once more, evaluation of this treatment is extremely important (see Chapter 7).

SUPPLEMENTARY TREATMENTS

Any child who has psychological problems, be they emotional, behavioral, or intellectual, may have other problems as well. Such children may need speech therapy, physical therapy, or a special diet; they may need just one of these supplemental treatments or they may need several of them. A general discussion of how to evaluate such supplemental treatments is given in Chapter 7.

All of the treatments described in this chapter have been presented as though they were separate treatment approaches always prescribed one by one. In fact, however, treatment approaches are often combined in order to meet several different needs of the child and/or family. For instance, probably the most typical treatment offered by child guidance clinics is for the child to be seen in individual psychotherapy by a psychiatrist while the parents are seen by a social worker for either individual or couples therapy.

Furthermore, it is becoming more and more common for therapists to utilize a mixture of psychotherapeutic and behavioral approaches, emphasizing one or the other depending on the specific client and the specific psychological difficulties involved. This chapter has not discussed these possible combination approaches. By viewing each aspect of a recommended treatment program separately, and thus by evaluating each separately, parents should be able to come to a reasonable understanding of any combination-treatment approach.

As a closing note to this chapter, it should be stressed that the above descriptions of treatments do not attempt to evaluate any of these treatments. The next chapter is devoted to evaluation. Hopefully, the present chapter has given parents enough familiarity with the kinds of treatments that might be recommended so that the following discussion of treatment evaluation will be meaningful and helpful to them.

> Alice laughed. "There's no use trying," she said:
> "one *can't* believe impossible things."
> "I daresay you haven't had much practice," said
> the Queen. "When I was your age, I always did it for
> half-an-hour a day. Why, sometimes I've believed as
> as many as six impossible things before breakfast."
>
> *Through the Looking-Glass*

How Do I Evaluate a Treatment Recommended for My Child?

CHAPTER 7

Before beginning to discuss specific evaluation procedures for specific treatment recommendations, it might help to put the issue of treatment for mental health problems into a larger perspective. As a scientific endeavor, the investigation of psychological processes underlying psychological difficulties is very young. This endeavor had its essential beginning in the late 1800s with Sigmund Freud being the best-known figure of that time. There were, of course, many writers from earlier times who discussed psychological issues, the Greek tragedians and biblical sources being notable examples, but these writings reflected the personal beliefs of the authors and were not based on the scientific method of systematic observation and variation. Thus, scientific investigation of those fundamental psychological processes relevant to psychological disturbance is no more than one hundred years old. And even this is an overestimate. Until the late 1940s, many procedures in psychological investigation were not very sophisticated, and it is now difficult to accept many of the findings of earlier studies due to what would now be seen as their procedural inadequacies. In fact, much of our actual working base of scientific understanding about the cause and treatment of psychological problems is little more than a generation old.

In addition to the youthfulness of psychology as a science, our understanding of mental health problems has been limited by the inherent complexity of the subject matter. Human behavior, with all its richness of thought and emotion, is very difficult to understand. At the moment, much more is understood about the principles and organization of the physical world than about the principles and organization of the human mind. Our knowledge of human behavior has increased tremendously during this century, but we have a very long way to go.

Without a precise and comprehensive understanding of fundamental psychological processes, the treatment of mental health problems will be more confusing and less predictable than any of us, professionals or clients, would like. There will be disagreement among professionals about what type of treatment approach is most effective; the discussion in this chapter will describe some of these disagreements as they presently exist. There will be treatment recommendations that are inadequate for the problem at hand. There will be treatment strategies that will seem adequate initially, but will not be effective in the long run. It is unfortunate that these things are the way they are. It would be much more pleasant to report that as mental health professionals, we are all in agreement, can recognize problems clearly, and can treat these problems effectively.

Perhaps someday in the future, this ideal world will exist. At the moment, it does not. Because it does not, parents will need to be actively involved in evaluating treatment recommendations that they receive from mental health professionals. This does not mean that parents should cease to trust and respect mental health professionals. It does mean that given our present state of knowledge we can take very little for granted and that to insure the best treatment for any child, both professionals and parents need to think carefully, work hard, and combine their knowledge about the child. On many occasions, such an approach will severely tax the ingenuity and patience of both professionals and parents. Unfortunately, this is simply the price we have to pay for excellence in mental health care. I believe that the alternative, the passive parent accepting everything the professional says without question, runs the risk, of the highest cost of all — inadequate and ineffective treatment.

A NOTE ON OBTAINING "SECOND OPINIONS"

At various times throughout this chapter, parents will be advised that obtaining a second opinion is an alternative they should consider. Since many parents will not be familiar with this procedure or may feel uncomfortable about it, some discussion would seem warranted.

In general, a second opinion is to be sought whenever parents are dissatisfied with the evaluation, treatment recommendation, or treatment their child is receiving *and* when this dissatisfaction had been discussed with the current professional but without an agreement having been reached between parents and professional. Thus, the first response to dissatisfaction should be to discuss it with the current professional; if this discussion fails to alter the parents' feelings, then obtaining a second opinion should be considered. If parents decide to obtain a second opinion, they should inform the first professional of their decision.

Ideally, this second professional should not be professionally associated with the first professional. Practically, this may be difficult. In a small town, for example, most mental health professionals will know each other; many of them may even work together upon occasion. If a second professional truly independent of the original professional is difficult to find, the parent can ask that the second professional conduct his or her evaluation without knowledge of the opinion of the first professional. Most professionals who are being consulted for a second opinion will be glad to do this, as they understand that the parent needs a second assessment of the child that is not biased by the findings of the first assessment.

Having sought and obtained a second opinion, parents have to decide how to respond to this additional information. There are a variety of possible situations that might occur. Consider the following examples.

1. First professional recommends X treatment; parents think Y treatment would be better; second professional recommends Y treatment. In this case, the parents will probably agree to follow the second professional's recommendation and decide to regard this person as "their" mental health professional. They will probably not return to the first professional, although they should notify the first professional of their decision. It should be noted that this sequence of events does not necessarily mean that X treatment is "wrong" and Y treatment is "right." It does mean that the parents will be more comfortable with Y treatment and, probably, with working with the second professional. This increased comfort can be an important contribution to the effectiveness of any treatment.

2. First professional recommends X treatment; parents think Y treatment would be better; second professional recommends X treatment. The parents in this situation have a difficult decision to make. They have two recommendations for X, but they continue to think Y is best. Do they continue to seek other opinions, hoping to find a professional who will recommend Y?
3. First professional recommends X treatment; parents think Y treatment would be better; second professional recommends Z treatment. Again, the parents are confronted with a difficult decision. Do they continue to seek other opinions?

There are no easy answers to the dilemmas presented in examples 2 and 3. On the one hand, parents have the right to seek as many opinions as they want. On the other hand, parents do not want to become "doctor shoppers," going from one mental health professional to another, endlessly seeking the treatment they want, and delaying their child's receiving any kind of care at all. Parents caught in the dilemmas illustrated in examples 2 and 3 will need to consider very carefully what they should do. They may, for example, feel that in a situation similar to that of example 2, they need to assess the reputations and independence of the two professionals they have consulted. If both have good professional reputations and are quite independent of one another, then the parents may decide to go ahead with the recommended treatment and work with whichever one of the two professionals the family prefers. The parents making this decision would be acknowledging that their preference for Y treatment is unlikely to receive professional support and that their preference may therefore have been in error. In situations resembling either examples 2 or 3, parents may want to discuss their dilemma with some trusted and respected family member or friend. Or they may ask either, or both, of the professionals involved to recommend reading material that the parents can consult in order to understand better the treatment(s) being recommended. Throughout this process, the parents should feel free to discuss with both professionals the feelings they (the parents) are having and why they are finding it difficult to make their decision.

The above discussion should not give parents a misleading impression. Only a few parents would ever find themselves confronting the types of situations described in examples 2 and 3. It is important, however, for all parents to know that they can seek additional professional opinions when they feel a need for this and to have some idea about the kinds of information that they might get from such additional consultation.

TREATMENT RECOMMENDATION: NO TREATMENT

A parent who receives the recommendation of no treatment will want to inquire carefully about the evidence upon which the professional has based this recommendation. If this evidence seems convincing to the parents, then they will probably feel vastly relieved and should feel that they were conscientious in checking out what appeared to be a problem. If, on the other hand, the evidence is not convincing to the parents, and they continue to believe that their child has a psychological problem, then the parents will want to obtain the opinion of a second mental health professional to see if this second opinion will agree with the first.

TREATMENT RECOMMENDATION: MODIFICATION OF PARENTAL EXPECTATIONS

In evaluating the recommendation that parental expectations need to change, the following outline indicates the major questions that a parent should ask.

BEFORE TREATMENT

1. Does it seem reasonable that unrealistic expectations on your part are an important part of the difficulties that you are experiencing with your child?
2. If not, obtain a second opinion.
3. If so, engage in treatment.

DURING TREATMENT

4. After a while, ask yourself if your expectations are changing.
5. If expectations are not changing, discuss this with the professional. His or her approach to changing parental expectations may have to be changed.
6. If your expectations are changing, has this reduced the difficulties with your child that first brought you to the mental health facility?
7. If expectations are changing, but the child's difficulties appear to be continuing, discuss this with the professional. Additional or different treatment may be necessary.

8. If your expectations are changing and the child's difficulties are being reduced, then treatment is working and the recommendation was appropriate.

The first three questions are directed at the initial decision—to engage in treatment or not—that parents have to make. In order to make this initial decision, they should keep two things in mind. First, they need to be convinced that the recommendation is a good one. For them to be convinced of this, they need to examine the evidence for the conclusion that they have unrealistic expectations that are creating difficulties for the child. Thus, parents need to ask themselves if at least some of the child's apparent problems could, in fact, really be a reflection of unrealistic expectations on their part. If it seems reasonable that unrealistic expectations could be an important part of their difficulties with their child, then the recommendation will seem appropriate. If, however, it does not seem reasonable that unrealistic expectations could account for a large part of their difficulties with their child, then they should obtain a second opinion.

Now, it should be noted, this initial part of the parents' evaluation of the treatment recommendation may not be as easy as it sounds. It is not a very pleasant experience for parents to be told that their expectations— and not the child's behavior—are the primary basis of the child's apparent difficulties. Indeed—and this will apply to many of the evaluations of treatment we will discuss in this chapter—it is not pleasant for parents to hear that they are in *any* way involved in creating their child's problem.

It often comes as a distinctly unwelcome surprise when parents hear from a mental health professional that they, as well as the child, will have to change in order to reduce the child's difficulties. Sometimes the unpleasant nature of this communication can result in parents taking a defensive stance that is unrealistic and will not help the child. Parents might deny that they have anything to do with the child's problem and can then act on this denial by avoiding the mental health professional who indicated that they are involved. On the other hand, parental behaviors are sometimes seen as the basis of a child's problem when, in fact, these behaviors have little to do with the problem at hand. How are the parents to know whether they are involved in the creation of their child's problem or not? How can parents avoid being defensive and yet also avoid accepting an inappropriate treatment recommendation?

There are, unfortunately, no easy answers to these questions, but there are some general guidelines that might help. Parents should attempt to be as open, receptive, and nondefensive as possible when discussing treatment recommendations. If, for example, the mental health professional focuses on the need to change parental expectations, parents should try very hard to avoid their initial defensive feelings of "Oh, no, that can't be the problem." Parents should try to assess the entire situation as objectively as possible. If a mental health professional focuses on parental expectations, parents should consider very seriously that their expectations may be an important factor in the child's apparent difficulties. To make an objective assessment, they will want to discuss the matter carefully with the mental health professional. They may also want to discuss this with trusted friends as well. After this serious consideration, parents will need to make their own decision. If it appears likely to them that parental expectations may be involved, then they can evaluate the treatment recommendation as a reasonable one. If, however, after the most objective consideration they can make, it seems quite unlikely that parental expectations are a significant factor in their child's problems, then they will want to obtain a second opinion.

The second issue that parents should keep in mind when evaluating a recommendation that they change their expectations is that any treatment to change these expectations probably will be of relatively brief duration, probably will not cost them a large amount of time or money, and should not significantly delay obtaining other types of treatment if it turns out that other types of treatment are needed. Thus, as long as the recommendation seems fairly reasonable and the anticipated duration of treatment is short, parents should probably go ahead and engage in the recommended discussions aimed at changing their expectations about the child's behavior.

The last five questions address parental concerns during treatment. After parents have worked for a while with a professional on changing their expectations, they should ask themselves if their expectations are changing. If they are not, then the professional's approach may not be working and this needs to be discussed with the professional. If expectations are changing, the parents need to ask themselves if this change has reduced their difficulties with their child. If these difficulties are not being reduced, then the professional needs to know this and may have to change or add to the treatment approach. If parental expectations are changing and difficulties with the child are being reduced, then the treatment is working and the recommendation was highly appropriate.

This discussion should make it clear that the task of evaluating a recommendation and the treatment deriving from this recommendation is a fairly complicated endeavor for the parent. Behind its complications, however, there are two very simple and straightforward principles that are fundamental throughout the material presented in this chapter.

1. *Use your common sense. Upon your best consideration, recommendations and treatments should seem reasonable to you.*
2. *The proof of the pudding is in the eating. The best evidence for the effectiveness of a treatment is that it works for you and for your child.*

Parents should keep these two principles in mind as they read the rest of this chapter.

TREATMENT RECOMMENDATION: PSYCHOTHERAPY

In Chapter 6, a variety of theories about and forms of psychotherapy were described. This section of the present chapter considers the effectiveness of psychotherapy and suggests some guidelines for parents to follow in evaluating a recommendation for psychotherapy. It should be noted that only three major forms of psychotherapy—individual, group, and family— are discussed specifically. The other two forms described in Chapter 6 can, for the purposes of the present discussion, be considered as subsumed by these major categories, with play therapy being a type of individual psychotherapy and couples therapy being a type of family therapy.

How Successful Is Psychotherapy?

Perhaps the best statement about the general success of psychotherapy as a treatment for mental health problems can be taken from an acknowledged expert in the field of psychotherapy research, Allen E. Bergin. Bergin states, "It now seems apparent that psychotherapy, as practiced over the past 40 years, has had an average effect that is modestly positive."[1] This means that, taken as a whole, people who enter psychotherapy are likely to receive some slight benefit from this treatment. Most importantly, how-

---

[1] Allen E. Bergin, "The Evaluation of Therapeutic Outcomes," in *Handbook of Psychotherapy and Behavior Change: An Empirical Analysis*, edited by Allen E. Bergin and Sol L. Garfield (New York: John Wiley and Sons, 1971), p. 263.

ever, Bergin has added a vital qualification to this finding. He indicates that a closer examination of the available evidence on the effectiveness of psychotherapy suggests that not all people in psychotherapy receive this modest benefit. In fact, Bergin's analysis shows that a number of people who engage in psychotherapy get *much better,* but that a number of other people get *much worse.* Thus, there is no simple way to view psychotherapy. Its general effect is for modest improvement, but it seems capable of providing either significantly beneficial or harmful results depending on the specific client and specific therapist.

What determines whether psychotherapy for a specific individual will be helpful is not well understood. At the moment, it looks as though one important factor may be the "match" between therapist and client. Some therapists seem to work very well with some clients; with other clients, these same therapists may not be so effective. Unfortunately, we are not able to specify in advance what characteristics of therapist and client are associated with good or bad "matches." Theoretical orientation of the therapist may be involved, some clients working better with psychoanalysts, others with interpersonally oriented therapists, and still others with client-centered therapists. The client's problem may be an essential feature: some therapists seem to be good at working with people who have a certain type of problem, but not very effective in working with other people with different types of problems. Or personality characteristics may be involved: personality "matches" and "clashes" are everyday occurrences, as well as possible therapeutic factors. Until we are better able to specify the exact therapist and client characteristics that create effective psychotherapy, parents are well advised to become acquainted with a number of types of therapy and, if possible, with several different possible therapists. This familiarity may allow them to make more accurate judgments about which specific therapist is going to work best with them and/or their child.

INDIVIDUAL PSYCHOTHERAPY

Levitt reports that research on psychotherapy with children has generally found an improvement rate of around 80 percent.[2] This rate, while sounding rather high, is not, however, significantly better than the improvement rate for children who were offered treatment but did not engage in it. Thus, there is no solid evidence that psychotherapy with children leads,

[2]Eugene E. Levitt, "Research on Psychotherapy with Children," in Bergin and Garfield, *Handbook,* pp. 474-94.

in general, to better outcomes for children than no psychotherapy at all. However, depending on the specific child and the specific therapist, both improvement and deterioration have been found following psychotherapy. Thus, the effectiveness of psychotherapy with children appears similar to that of psychotherapy with adults: either beneficial or harmful results can be brought about, depending on the individual client and the specific therapist.

GROUP THERAPY

There is relatively little published research evidence concerning the effectiveness of chidlren's groups. One review article, however, has concluded that the "available evidence . . . is inconclusive, but nonetheless discouraging."[3] While some of the studies reviewed found that group therapy with children led to improvement, a similar number found that no improvement was obtained. Furthermore, a few studies indicated that group therapy can have harmful consequences, with the children getting worse rather than getting better or staying the same. At the present time, then, group therapy with children has not demonstrated general effectiveness. On the other hand, depending on the specific client, the specific therapist, and, perhaps, the specific type of group, improvement or deterioration is possible.

FAMILY THERAPY

Family therapy is a new and increasingly popular form of psychotherapy. In this therapy, the therapist (or therapists, as is not infrequent) see all of the members of a family during a group session. Sometimes very young children are not included, although sometimes they are, and on occasion, other relatives (grandparents, aunts, uncles) besides the primary family members are included when it is thought that they are involved in family problems. Family therapists tend to be fairly active therapists, more intrusive and directive than they might be when seeing a client on an individual basis. This increased activity reflects the practical fact that not much is likely to be accomplished at a family session if the family is left to continue in its usual and, by now habitual, interactions. Such usual interactions would include, for example, some members not talking, other talking at length, some blaming others, others defending themselves, and so on. In order to assist family members to work toward the therapeutic

---

[3]Abramowitz, Christine V., "The Effectiveness of Group Psychotherapy with Children," *Archives of General Psychiatry*, 1976, 33, p. 321.

goals, rather than simply continue nonbeneficial interactions, most family therapists find that they have to become fairly directive.

Although family therapy is becoming a widely used technique in working with children and their parents, there is little research evidence on its effectiveness. We have the somewhat peculiar situation of a great many theoretical writings on family therapy, and not nearly so many well-conducted studies of its effectiveness. Thus, at the moment, it cannot be said of family therapy that "it works"; on the other hand, it cannot be said that it doesn't

Evaluating Psychotherapy

From the preceding review of the effectiveness of psychotherapy, parents should realize that it is very important for them to evaluate carefully any recommendation that they or their child engage in psychotherapy as a treatment for the child's or family's difficulties. The need for evaluation is created by the findings on individual and group therapy (findings that also may be obtained in future research on family therapy): some people can be helped by some therapies, while others can be harmed. Thus, for many people, psychotherapy will not be a neutral event and, therefore, must be carefully evaluated. In evaluating psychotherapy (whether it be for parent or child, and whether it be individual, group, or family), the following guidelines should be helpful.

1. Every treatment recommendation is based on the mental health professional's identification and understanding of the characteristics of the child's problem. *Do the parents agree with the professional's identification of the problem?* For example, the therapist may feel that Johnny's major problem is that he lacks self-confidence. Do the parents agree that this is a major problem for Johnny? If they do not agree with the identified problem, they should seek a second opinion *regardless* of the treatment recommendation that is given. Agreement between parents and professional on the problem must precede making treatment plans.

2. Once parents and professional agree on the problem, parents should consider whether the treatment (in this case, psychotherapy) appears to be suitable for helping the child overcome his problem. For example, do the parents think it that Johnny, by talking with the therapist once a week, will become more self-confident? If it is unclear to the parents how

the recommended treatment is supposed to help the identified problem, then the parents will want the therapist to explain this relationship in detail. *Parents should not agree to any recommended treatment until they think it is reasonable to expect that this treatment will help solve the identified problem.*

3. Before agreeing to engage in a treatment, parents should inquire as to *what possible harmful effects might result.* One possible harmful effect that must always be considered is that psychotherapy will not benefit the child, the child will thus get older without any improvement in the problem, and thus the child's problem will become more and more difficult for both the child and other family members. Apart from this general possibility, however, there may be specific harmful effects. For example, if Johnny is given to brooding about himself, a psychotherapy that concentrates on Johnny's talking about himself may run the risk of increasing his brooding and his feeling badly about himself. Mental health professionals should always be willing to discuss seriously any possible harm that might come to the child from the recommended treatment. Parents who feel that the professional whom they are seeing is not taking the possibility of harm seriously enough should consult another mental health professional.

4. *Assess the benefit-harm ratio.* Parents need to make sure that professionals state their estimate of the likelihood that the child will be helped by psychotherapy and their estimate of the likelihood that the child will be harmed by psychotherapy.

$$\frac{\text{Possible benefit}}{\text{Possible harm}}$$

Before agreeing to engage in a treatment, the parents must be convinced that the possible benefit clearly outweighs any possible harm.

5. *What procedures will the professional use to evaluate the effects of the treatment?* If at this point the parents feel that the professional has a good grasp of their child's problems, has given a convincing explanation of how psychotherapy will alleviate these problems, and has persuaded them that the possible benefit outweighs the possible harm, then parents are probably well advised to accept the recommendation for psychotherapy-if, in addition, the professional can specify the procedures to be used to evaluate the child's progress. This additional criterion is very important. It is simply not sufficient to recommend and implement a treatment, but never bother to document whether this treatment is, in fact, having the

desired effects. Professionals should state to parents their initial estimate of how long psychotherapy will be necessary for the child and at what point and how they will assess the effects of psychotherapy. There are many ways in which this might be done. For example:

A. Estimated therapy time might be one year, with periodic assessments of the child's behavior every three months. The professional might stipulate that if the child shows no improvement after six months, he or she will want to consider changing the treatment the child is receiving—either modifying the approach in psychotherapy, recommending supplementary experiences, or recommending changing from psychotherapy to some other treatment approach.
B. Estimated therapy time might be three months, with an assessment only at this time.

A general rule of thumb that the parent might follow is that with longer estimated therapy times, more intervening assessments will be necessary, while with shorter estimated therapy time only one assessment (at the end of therapy) may be necessary.

The exact assessment schedule proposed will of course vary widely depending on the specific child, the specific therapist, and the specific problem. The schedule as a whole, however, should seem reasonable to the parents. They should not expect that the schedule can be rigidly adhered to without exception—it might well be necessary to revise estimated therapy time (either upward or downward) in the course of treatment. However, parents should expect that the therapist will give general estimates that in general will prove accurate. They should also expect the therapist to be committed to evaluating the effects of the therapeutic interventions. If the therapist will not discuss evaluation procedures with the parents, or if the procedures that are discussed seem terribly inappropriate, they should consider going to another professional. Table 7-1 provides some examples of good and bad evaluation procedures.

These guidelines for evaluation are not foolproof. With the best intentions and maximum effort, a therapist may recommend psychotherapy, the parents may accept, and the child may get no better, or may even get worse. If this should happen, no doubt everyone involved will feel badly—everyone will have failed to bring about the desired benefit to the child. Most importantly, though, everyone will know that they did their very best to help the child. Secure in this knowledge, parents and professional can go on to consider alternative treatments without blaming each other or themselves. Individuals will be to blame, however,

TABLE 7-1
Examples of Good and Bad Evaluation Procedures Planned by Therapists to Evaluate the Effectiveness of Their Treatment.

Good Procedures	Bad Procedures
1. *Highly specific.* "I'll have another professional give Mark these achievement tests again and I'll obtain a detailed report from his teacher. This should let us know how his learning is coming along."	1. *Vague.* "Well, I always know when my clients are improving."
2. *Appropriate timing.* "I'll come and observe Linda at home and at school at the end of every three months of therapy. This should let us know how she's progressing."	2. *Inappropriate Timing.* "I think therapy will take several years. At the end of therapy, I'll be glad to evaluate Linda's progress.
3. *Does not depend solely on self-report of the client, but utilizes other information as well.* "I'll have Claude keep a diary of his feelings and, in addition, I'd like you to keep a record of his extracurricular activites, including times when he has friends over to the house. Also, I'll make periodic observations at the school. All of this together should give us a pretty good idea of how Claude feels about himself and of how he's relating to other people."	3. *Relies on self-report of the client without gathering other information.* "I'll be sure to ask Claude every once in a while how he feels."

if an unreasonable treatment is offered and accepted, and if evaluation procedures are too casual and/or infrequent. Professionals have an obligation to make their best effort to provide the best possible treatment, and parents have an obligation to see to it that they do.

TREATMENT RECOMMENDATION:
BEHAVIOR THERAPY

In Chapter 6 some types of behavior therapy techniques were described. This section discusses the effectiveness of behavior therapy and suggests some guidelines for parents to follow in evaluating a recommendation for behavior therapy. It should be noted that behavior therapy can be conducted with individuals, groups, or families. In working with children, most behavior therapists also work with their parents.

As a psychologist, I am almost bound to be biased in favor of behavior therapy. Behavior therapy is an approach to therapy that has been created primarily by psychologists (although J. Wolpe, the founder of systematic densensitization, is a physician and thus a striking exception to this generalization). Behavior therapy is derived from principles of learning, principles that have been established by psychologists doing basic research on learning. These principles are then applied to problem behaviors in an effort to change them. Since most behavior therapists were trained as psychologists, they have been committed to research and have conducted more systematic evaluations of their techniques than has been done with the other nonphysical approaches to psychological problems.

This emphasis on research has led to a state of affairs today in which scarcely anyone would question that behavior therapy can be successful with specific problems, including, for example: phobic behaviors (avoiding feared objects, such as avoiding school), enuresis (bedwetting), increasing self-help skills (washing oneself, making one's bed), decreasing self-destructive behavior (particularly in psychotic children), and decreasing disruptive behavior in the classroom. There is some controversy about exactly how a specific behavior therapy technique produces a specific effect,[4] and there is some question about the kind of research that has been conducted.[5] In spite of these theoretical and methodological controversies,

---

[4]For example, while as a psychologist I may be biased in favor of behavior therapy, as a psychologist who thinks in terms of social psychological theory rather than learning theory I tend to explain the effectiveness of behavior therapy techniques on grounds differing from those invoked by most current practitioners. Increasingly, studies are being conducted that attempt to sort out the basic psychological processes by which behavior therapy techniques have their effects.

[5]In all too many cases, a single-subject experiment has been used. This single-subject approach does offer more control than the case study method used by psychoanalysts and more traditional psychotherapists. In the case study method, the therapist simply reports on his or her ongoing treatment of a person. There is no attempt to gather more scientifically acceptable evidence to indicate that one sort of intervention has led to one sort of behavior on the part of the client. In a typical single-subject study, the behavior therapist collects (baseline) data on how the client is behaving prior to treatment (phase A). The therapist then institutes behavior therapy and evaluates the client's behavior (phase B). The next step is to stop the therapeutic intervention and evaluate the client's behavior (phase A). Then the behavior therapist introduces the therapy once more and evaluates the client's behavior (phase B). This is called an ABAB design. If the problem behavior is infrequent during B periods and frequent during A periods, then we have some confidence that the therapist's intervention is affecting the client's behavior in the desired manner. Unfortunately, however, single-subject

however, there is no doubt that behavior therapy represents at the present moment the approach to the psychological treatment of psychological problems that has the most documented evidence of effectiveness.

Most psychotherapists would not dispute this evidence. Some would, however, question whether it is appropriate to address therapy to "simple" behavior problems. Psychotherapists have argued that psychological problems tend to be more complex than simply, for example, avoiding school. They might suggest in a specific case that the child's relationship with her parents need to be considered in detail and improved, and that simply increasing her school attendance won't solve her "real" problem. In other words, if behavior therapy gets the child to go to school more often, her "real" problem in relating to her parents will crop up again in some other area, perhaps in an inability to make good grades in school.

I do not wish this book to become an extended discussion of the merits of psychotherapy versus those of behavior therapy, but having indicated the type of objection that is likely to be raised to behavior therapy, I should indicate the response a behavior therapist might give:

"OK, first of all you make the assumption that I would simply try to increase school attendance without attending to any of the reasons why the child avoided school in the first place. That would not be good behavior therapy. I would first conduct a functional analysis of the child's behavior, where I would seek to find the relationships between environmental events and the child's behavior. This analysis might discover, for instance, that the child only stays home when the mother is home. If this were found, it would suggest that the relationship with the mother is critical, and that the focus of the behavior therapy should be on having the mother spend more out-of-school time with the child. Thus, I too would work on the child's relationships with others, but in a more specific, behaviorally oriented manner."

At this point, the psychotherapist might respond:

"But you're making it too simple. The child's problem with the mother isn't simply one of spending more fun time with the mother. The child is deeply dependent on the mother, but also resents her greatly. This ambivalence leads the child to have destructive fantasies about getting rid of the

---

designs "prove" the case only for that single individual. In order to demonstrate the technique's effectiveness for wider use with many individuals, studies have to be done examining the response of many individuals to the specific treatment. These multiple-subject studies are beginning to be done more frequently by behavior therapists, and evidence collected in these studies has in general supported the effectiveness of behavior therapy techniques.

mother, as well as to fear that these fantasies might come true, thus needing to stay home to make sure that they don't."

At this point, the dialogue in our example has broken down. The behavior therapist might respond by saying that the behavior therapist could work on fantasies if these were the problem, but this answer would not satisfy the psychotherapist either. We have reached a true impasse. The psychotherapist will tend to take an intrapsychic approach, concentrating on the feelings of the child. The behavior therapist will tend to take a situational approach, concentrating on those environmental events that may cause the child's feelings. This is probably a true difference between these therapies and one that no amount of research will easily resolve. Psychotherapists will be willing to grant that behavior therapy techniques work with certain problems, but they will continue to argue that in general these problems grow out of more central psychological conflicts that behavior therapy does not affect.

Fortunately, not all parents will be confronted with such an ideological dispute. Increasingly in recent years, therapists have begun to combine psychotherapy and behavior therapy and use techniques from both approaches. Furthermore, recent research suggests that with well trained and highly experienced therapists, psychotherapy and behavior therapy tend to produce similar beneficial results. It is still possible, however, for parents to be advised that only one type of therapy is being recommended and that this one type is the only type of therapy that they should consider as being appropriate for their child. In such instances, parents would benefit from having some information about how to compare the probable effectiveness of behavior therapy versus psychotherapy.

To make this comparison, parents can examine the pervasiveness of the child's problem. If the child's difficulty seems to be fairly specific and circumscribed—limited, for example, to interactions with one person, or to one place, or to one activity, or involving just one behavior—then behavior therapy may be the more appropriate treatment. If, on the other hand, the child's problems seem quite diffuse—occurring in interactions with many people, in many places, during many activities, involving many behaviors—then psychotherapy may be more suitable.

In addition, there is a certain practical distinction between the two approaches. Behavior therapy typically takes considerably less time than traditional psychotherapy. If a behavior therapist fails to make sufficient progress, this is usually reasonably evident (given the behavior therapist's emphasis on gathering data about the behavior being addressed) fairly early on. Psychotherapy, however, tends to deemphasize immediate behavior change (so that even if progress is being made, it may not be evident), and it takes longer. Thus if the major possible harmful effect in therapy with children is that the child might get older without improving, then behavior therapy is the safer choice. A behavior therapy program can fail and the child will not have gotten that much older. This child can then receive psychotherapy, and the chances for success in psychotherapy should not have changed much. If, on the other hand, psychotherapy is tried first and fails, its failure may not be apparent until years later. At this point, the child will have had problems for many more years, and the chances for engaging in a successful behavior therapy program may well have decreased. On these grounds, it can be argued that behavior therapy is frequently a good approach to try first.

Evaluating Behavior Therapy

Parental procedures for evaluating behavior therapy are the same as for evaluating psychotherapy, and these procedures are outlined below. It should be noted that evaluation of the progress made in behavior therapy is usually easier than evaluating progress made in psychotherapy; as noted previously, the behavior therapist is more likely than the psychotherapist to "build in" readily understandable evaluation procedures into therapy.

1. Do the parents agree with the professional's identification of the problem? Parents and professional must agree on the characteristics of the child's problem before treatment can proceed. If this agreement does not develop, parents should seek a second opinion.
2. Once parents and professional agree on the problem, parents need to understand how the recommended treatment is supposed to help the identified problem. If this understanding cannot be obtained, parents should seek a second opinion.
3. The professional should explain to the parents the possible harmful effects of the therapy.
4. Parents should assess the benefit-harm ratio. Before agreeing to proceed with therapy, the parents must be convinced that the possible benefit outweighs any possible harm.
5. The professional should state to the parents his or her initial estimate of how long behavior therapy will be necessary for the child, and at what point and how the effects of the therapy will be assessed.

Only when parents and the professional understand each other and are in agreement on the above five issues should parents agree to have their child engage in the recommended treatment.

TREATMENT RECOMMENDATION: CHILD-REARING COUNSELING OR PARENT EFFECTIVENESS TRAINING

Both child-rearing counseling and parent effectiveness training (PET) can be classified as parent counseling. They differ in how they are implemented. Child-rearing counseling typically takes place between a professional and one family, while parent effectiveness training typically involves a child-rearing expert speaking with a group of parents. There is some evidence that parent counseling does improve parent-child interactions, but a great deal more research remains to be done in order to ascertain the best methods of parent counseling and the types of problems that are most likely to be helped. At present, we can say that parent counseling appears to be a promising approach to at least some problems. The parent considering a recommendation for parent counseling should utilize the general evaluative procedures outlined in more detail in the discussions of evaluating psychotherapy and behavior therapy. These procedures can be summarized as follows:

1. Does the parent agree that parent counseling may help reduce the child's difficulties?
2. What are the possible harmful effects? Do the potential benefits outweigh the potential harm?
3. What are the evaluation procedures the professional will use to determine whether parent counseling has obtained the desired goals?

TREATMENT RECOMMENDATION: SUPPORTIVE THERAPY

Supportive therapy is a type of therapeutic approach where no change is sought, but where maintenance of the person's current level of psychological functioning is the goal. Such support may be helpful in a variety of situations—for example, following a more intensive therapeutic experience, or for families facing long-term problems that cannot be significantly changed, or for parents and children who need to "get through" a crisis period before they can consider working on behavioral or emotional changes. Supportive therapy could be conducted from either a psychotherapeutic or behavioral orientation. There is little evidence concerning the specific effectiveness of supportive therapy. We do not know if it is effective, but then again, we do not know that it is ineffective. When supportive therapy is recommended (for the parents, the child, or both), parents should follow the evaluation procedures outlined for evaluating psychotherapy and behavior therapy, but should keep in mind that the desired effect is to provide support for the client(s), not to effect change.

TREATMENT RECOMMENDATION: SPECIAL EDUCATION

In this discussion, *special education* will refer to any educative technique that is in addition to or different from regular classroom experiences in a regular school. This is the same definition that was used in Chapter 6. The basic steps in evaluating a recommedation for special education are quite similar to the procedures discussed for evaluating previous treatment approaches, but there are some special aspects concerning educative treatment that need to be explained.

1. Does the parent agree that the child's problem consists of or is worsened by a difficulty in learning or difficulties in other school-related behaviors (for example, paying attention in class, interacting with peers and/or teachers)? If special education is the only treatment that is recommended, then the parent should be convinced that the assistance offered by special education will solve the problem that brought the parent and child to the mental health facility. For example, special education may well be the primary treatment for a child whose major problems in learning and/or social behavior occur in the school setting, but special education alone may not be enough for a very fearful child who is doing poorly in school and is very withdrawn and shy in all social situations. If parents feel that there are other problems that will not be solved by special education, they should indicate this to the professional and ask whether other or additional treatment recommendations should be made to meet these other problems.

If, on the other hand, special education is one of a number of treatment recommendations, the parent should ask the question, "Is there a need for my child to receive special education?" If the parent perceives such a need, the treatment recommendation will seem appropriate. If the parent does not perceive such a need, he or she should ask the professional why the recommendation for special education was made. In the latter case, professionals should be able to document why they believe a child's learning or other school-related behaviors need to be improved.

2. How will the specific special education program that is recommended assist the child? The parent should ask for some evidence from the professional that the specific type of educative program that is recommended has, in fact, demonstrated effectiveness with children who have school-related problems similar to their child's. To help parents understand how the specific program will help their child, parents may wish to observe the program as it works with other children. Before or during this observation (arrangements for which can be made by the mental health professional), parents can ask whether there are other children in the program whose psychological problems are similar to their child's and, if so, can observe the responses of such children to the educative program. If parents observe that children who have had problems reasonably similar to those of their child appear to be getting along well in the special educative program (for example, participating in classroom activities, getting along with teachers and peers, tackling learning tasks that appear challenging and yet not frustrating), then parents should regard the program favorably. In addition to observation, the parents will want to talk with the teachers involved in the special education program and get their views on the program they offer and the type of children they can help.

3. The parent should discuss with the professional, and the special education teachers as well, the possible harmful effects of the educative program being recommended. One rather common possible harmful effect is that the child will become labeled by other children as different (because the child attends a different class or different school). The labels used by other children can sometimes be quite vicious and can make children in special programs feel badly about themselves. The parent should ask if the education program takes any steps to try to reduce the possibility of the child's being labeled by other children. The parent should also inquire as to how rewarding the social relationships within the special education program are likely to be. If children can form good, satisfying relationships with other children in the program, they are much less likely to be hurt by children not in the program regarding them as different or calling them names.

4. Parents need to assess the benefit-harm ratio. For instance, it may be that a child in a special education program does run a certain risk of being

called names by children not in the program. If a specific child's need to improve his learning or other school-related behaviors is not very great, then this social risk may be too great and the parent may want to find out if there are other ways to obtain special education for the child (such as home tutoring) that will not incur this social risk. If, on the other hand, a certain child's need to improve her learning or other school-related behaviors is great, then the parent may decide that the risks the child will run if she does *not* enter the special education program (such risks as continued behavioral and/or learning problems in class, being called names by the other children anyway because of her difficulties in class, problems in learning the basic skills necessary to have an independent life in the society) are greater than the social harm she might incur if she enters the program. In this case, the benefits that may be obtained through improving the child's learning and/or school behaviors outweigh the possible harm that might occur, and the parents would want to accept the treatment recommendation.

5. The parent should inquire of the professional and of the special education teachers which procedures will be utilized to evaluate whether the special education is, indeed, improving the child's learning and/or school behaviors. Evaluation of the program's effectiveness is extremely important. If the child is not learning the desired new behaviors (for improved learning or other school behaviors), then alternative approaches must be considered. The parent should also inquire about the professional's plans to evaluate the child's *general* progress. A general evaluation of this sort is especially important when the child has been improving in the class. It is then important to know if this improvement has been sufficiently beneficial or if the child, even though improving in some areas, still has significant psychological difficulties. In the latter case, treatment approaches other than special education may be necessary in addition to, or in place of, the special education program.

TREATMENT RECOMMENDATION: MEDICATION

The use of medication to treat psychological problems of children is usually controversial. Some people will support the use of medication; others will not (see, for example, *Hyperactivity: Research, Theory, and Action* by D. Ross and S. Ross (New York: Wiley, 1976) for discussion of the controversy concerning the use of drugs to treat hyperactivity). Probably to take either extreme position is ill-advised. To put it simply: if a drug can help a child significantly, then the drug probably should be used; if a drug cannot help the child significantly, then the drug obviously should not be used. What is important is that the individual child, specific medication, and particular situation of the child be considered.

Let us assume that a parent has been advised to administer a medication to a child to help the child with a psychological problem. Here are some questions the parent should ask:

1. Do the parents agree with the professional's identification of the child's problems? This question is exactly the same one as has been discussed when evaluation procedures for psychological treatments were described. Parents and professionals must agree on the nature and characteristics of the child's problem before they can discuss treatment recommendations.

2. Is it reasonable to expect that by taking a medication, the child's problems will be reduced? In answering this question, the parent will have to consider carefully how the medication might be expected to affect the child's identified problem. If, for example, the parent and professional have agreed that a child is unhappy because the child does not get along with his or her peers, the parent will need to inquire of the professional how taking a medication could help the child get along with his or her peers. Or if the parent and professional believe the child is inattentive and too easily distracted and this causes the child to have difficulty in settling down and learning effectively, then the parent will need to inquire whether the medication that is recommended has been shown to increase children's attention span and decrease their tendency to be distracted. Thus, parents should ask the professional about the evidence for a link between the recommended medication and the child's problems. Only when this link has been demonstrated should the parent be willing to agree to having the medication administered to the child.

3. What possible harmful side effects might the medication produce? Before the administration of any medication to a child, the parent should inquire as to the side effects of the recommended medication. All medications do have side effects, and the probability of these side effects appearing to a significant degree must be understood by the parent.

4. What is the benefit-harm ratio? Parents need to discuss the following relationship with the professional recommending the medication.

$$\frac{\text{Potential benefits of medication}}{\text{Potential harmful side effects}}$$

As long as the potential benefits clearly outweigh the potential harm, then administration of the drug is a reasonable, medically sound procedure. If, however, the potential harmful side effects are greater than the potential benefit, then the medication should not be administered. In evaluating the benefit-harm ratio for medications, parents need adequate information on the medication(s) being discussed. Professionals should provide this information. If, for any reason, parents are dissatisfied with the information that the professional is providing them on a medication, parents can consult the *Physicians Desk Reference* (PDR), which is available in any good library. Most of the information in the *PDR* is supplied by the manufacturers of the drugs discussed and may not always have been verified by an independent assessment, but the information is good enough for the parent to get a general idea of what types of problems are helped by the medication and a specific idea of the side effects (these latter being listed in some detail).

5. What are the procedures the professional will utilize to test the effectiveness of the medication for the child? It is ill advised to administer a medication without a preplanned program to check on the effectiveness of the medication and the possible occurrence of any harmful side effects. This check must be systematic and stringent. It is not sufficient simply to say, "Well, give Carolyn these pills and let me know how she is coming along." Because evaluation of medication is so important and because this evaluation tends to be rather complex, the following example is offered. The details of administrating any specific medication will differ considerably from individual to individual, and so will the evaluation procedures employed. There should be, however, a sufficient number of similar principles involved in any evaluation so that the following example will be of some general assistance to parents.

Evaluating a Medication: An Example

Mark was brought to the clinic by his parents who were concerned about his behavior and about his lack of learning in school. A careful evaluation of Mark, including observations in both the home and school, revealed that he was, indeed, a hyperactive child: he was extremely energized, but in a diffuse, nonconstructive fashion; he was inattentive and very easily distracted in school; his behavior was disorganized and frequently highly aggressive, involving temper tantrums and outbursts in class. The professional suggested that Mark be given a specific medication to calm him down and increase his attention span. It was pointed out to the parents that while there is some possibility that this medication may decrease physical growth during childhood, Mark was quite a big child and thus there was less concern about Mark in regard to this possible side effect than there might be about some other children. Additionally, it was noted that some children do not react in the desired fashion to the medication, becoming more restless rather than less; or they may overreact, such that they are sedated (and may fall asleep) rather than simply being calmed. The parents felt that it was reasonable to think that if Mark were calmer and more attentive, he would be more manageable, feel better, and be able to learn better. They were concerned about the possibility of reducing Mark's physical growth, but felt that at the moment his psychological functioning was more important than some slight decrease in growth, especially since Mark was large for his age anyway. They also were concerned that Mark not react adversely to the medication.

The professional devised the following program for administration of the medication to Mark:

1. The first dosage to be given to Mark was based on previous research with the drug and Mark's physical size. A five-week trial period of administration was set up with the following features:

   a. The parents received an envelope for each day of the five weeks. All the envelopes contained pills that looked exactly alike. In fact, however, some of the pills contained the medication and some were simply sugar pills ("placebos"). Only the professional knew which was which, and thus the parents would not know when Mark received the medication rather than a placebo — and neither would Mark. This "double-blind" procedure was used to make sure that any changes in Mark's behavior were really due to the medication and not simply to the parents' or child's *belief* that the medication would change his behavior. Because neither Mark nor his parents knew when he was actually receiving medication, his teacher also could not know which days were "medication days" and which were "placebo days." This strategy prevented the teacher from treating Mark differently according to whether or not he had taken medication.
   b. Each day the parent and teacher kept track of Mark's behavior. There were three areas to be assessed:
      1. Attention span (how long Mark stayed at a specific task) and tendency to be distracted (how often Mark got out of his desk chair). These were the specific areas that the medication was supposed to improve.
      2. Mark's temper tantrums, aggressive behavior, and performance on school tasks. These were the behaviors that were to benefit from changes in 1.

3. How much Mark slept at night, how he felt in the morning, and whether he fell asleep during school. These concerned the adverse reactions that Mark might experience.

2. After five weeks, the professional evaluated Mark's behavior, looking at Mark's behavior when he actually had received the medication and when he had received a placebo. Depending on these data, the professional might reach any one of several conclusions:

   a. No effect of either medication or placebo. A higher dosage of the medication might be tried for another trial period.
   another trial period.
   b. Similar improvement under both medication and placebo. Since the placebo works as well as the medication, the medication is unnecessary and psychological procedures should be able to bring about improvement.
   c. More effect of the medication than of the placebo; no undesirable side effects. It would probably be recommended that Mark continue taking the medication.
   d. More effect of the medication than of the placebo, but Mark is falling asleep in class. Might then try lower dosage of the medication for a trial period.

If the data revealed result c — either now or after other trial periods — then all subsequent taking of the medication should be monitored. For instance, the professional might reinstitute double-blind procedures every three months. Monitoring of the child's behavior should continue throughout the period that he is taking the medication.

The essence of this complicated procedure is simply that a child should take a medication only when the medication has a clearly demonstratable positive effect. Parents should not agree to let the child take medication for any long period of time without some sort of evaluation procedures. If a professional recommends a drug, but is not prepared to evaluate its effects, I would strongly recommend that the parents go elsewhere and find a professional who is prepared to carefully assess the effects of the medication.

Let us suppose that an adequate evaluation has been done of the recommended medication and it has been clearly shown that the medication benefits the child. The child then begins to take the medication on a regular basis. The parent should be concerned about two issues during this medication phase. The first has already been mentioned above: it is very important that periodic checks be made of both the effectiveness of the drug and possible side effects. If at any point the harm from side effects begins to outweigh the beneficial effects of the medication, then the dosage level will have to be reduced or the child taken off the medication. Furthermore, if at any time the medication ceases to have its beneficial effects, then raising the dosage may be necessary and renewed checking on side effects will of course be necessary with increased dosage. It is not unusual for children (or adults) to develop a "tolerance" for a medication such that increased dosage levels become necessary if the medication is to continue having its effects. Also, if the drug ceases to have a clear drug-related — as opposed to placebo-related — effect, then it may be that the drug is no longer necessary at any dosage level and should be withdrawn completely. These are all fairly complex issues and can be evaluated only with good data made available through periodic checks on the medication's effects.

The second issue that parents need to attend to during the time the child takes a medication is also fairly complex. In essence, it is an issue that stems from the basic belief that except when absolutely necessary (for example, for certain physical conditions such as diabetes), no one wants a child (or an adult) to be taking any medication forever. This issue should be raised by parents once a drug evaluation study has proved the drug's usefulness: "How long do you expect my child will have to take this medication?" If the professional answers, "Forever," the parent may well want a second opinion to confirm or disconfirm this conclusion. If, as is more likely, the professional indicates that at some point the child will not have to take the medication any longer, the parents will want to inquire about the professional's plans for this.

In many problems with children, medication can serve as a temporary or supplementary therapeutic approach. The long-term goal with most children is to effect changes that are not solely drug-induced. For example, one approach with our example child Mark might be to utilize a medication initially so as to make it more possible to affect his behavior later through nonmedication approaches. Some hyperactive children are so disorganized that they cannot benefit immediately from nonphysical treatment programs. Some medications, when they are appropriately prescribed and evaluated, can make such children less easily distracted and more attentive to changes in their environment designed to help them maintain more appropriate behavior in the long run. Suppose, for example, that Mark's parents had developed the habit of only paying attention to him when he was hyperactive, thus rewarding him with attention for undesirable behavior. After he began taking the drug, Mark's parents might begin to work on rewarding him with their attention for desirable, nonhyperactive behaviors. Additionally, it might be that Mark's present school classroom is too full of distractions for Mark to concentrate, and so it would be desirable to place him in a less distracting classroom environment. These changes in parent behavior and school environment would be designed to facilitate Mark's becoming calmer and more attentive, with the long-term goal of withdrawing the medication so that Mark's new behaviors could be maintained by these other, nonmedication influences.

Thus, a careful program of drug administration for children should include plans for switching them off drug control of their behavior and onto control of their behavior by themselves and their everyday environment. This switching, however, cannot be counted on to occur by itself. The professional must plan from the very beginning to work toward that day when medication will no longer be required. Parents need to ask professionals if they are doing this. If the professional answers no, I strongly suggest that parents go elsewhere. Unless he or she is prepared to argue that the child will need the medication forever, the professional should be making plans to create a social and physical environment for the child that will both benefit the child and make it eventually unnecessary to take medication.

TREATMENT RECOMMENDATION: INPATIENT CARE

To have a child live away from home in order to provide mental health treatment is an enormously significant action. In order to discuss evaluation of such a recommendation, it may help to focus on two types of inpatient care: providing short-term treatment, and providing inpatient care for what is perceived to be a very long time. For both types of inpatient treatment, parents will want to keep in mind the guidelines that have been offered concerning evaluation of treatment recommendations. Before agreeing to any treatment recommendation:

1. Parents should agree with the professional's identification of the nature of the child's problems.
2. They should understand how the recommended treatment is supposed to help the child and/or family.
3. They should assess the possible harm that might be produced by the treatment.
4. They should assess the benefit-harm ratio.

5. They should be informed as to the evaluation procedures that the professional will utilize to keep track of the child's progress as the child engages in the recommended treatment.

Within this general framework, there are some more specific issues concerning inpatient care for children. The following discussion will address these specific issues.

Short-Term Inpatient Care

Short-term inpatient care may be provided in a variety of settings: psychiatric wards in general hospitals, psychiatric hospitals, group homes, schools for emotionally disturbed children. The time period involved may range from a few weeks to months to years. As long as the goal is to return the child to the community, it may be regarded as short-term for the purposes of this discussion.

When short-term inpatient care is recommended, the parents first need to make sure they agree with the professional's view of the nature and severity of the child's problems. Once agreement is reached on these issues, the parents should ask if there is any way to obtain the needed treatment through outpatient facilities. Parents should be sure to ask the professional why inpatient care is necessary rather than the forms of outpatient therapy that have been described previously in this book. Inpatient treatment is a very significant action and should be regarded as a last resort that one turns to only when outpatient approaches are not suitable. Having stated this, it also should be said that there are occasions when outpatient approaches are not suitable and an inpatient facility is needed. The most dramatic instances involve the possibility of children's injuring themselves or others. Less dramatic instances involve children who have not benefited from outpatient approaches and whose problems may be getting worse, or children whose families cannot cope with present levels of stress. Whatever the specific circumstances, the parents must be convinced that inpatient care is necessary and that outpatient treatment would not be sufficient.

If inpatient care as a general treatment approach appears reasonable to the parents, they will still need to ask about the specific treatments that will be conducted with the child. How long will the child probably need to be in the facility? Length of inpatient stay should always be justified in terms of the length of time it will take to have the child engage in specific treatments (such as psychotherapy, behavior therapy, education, etc.). What problems will be worked on while the child is staying in the facility and how will these problems be worked on? When considering specific treatments that will be offered in the hospital, the parents should follow the previously presented guidelines for evaluating treatments. Parents should agree to inpatient care for their child only when they are convinced that the specific treatments can reasonably be expected to help the child and that the length of time necessary to conduct these treatments seems appropriate.

Additionally, parents will want to inquire as to their role. Will they be included in the child's treatment through, for example, being seen at the facility for individual or group therapy? How will they be informed about the child's progress? Will they meet periodically with the professional in charge of their child's care? When and how often will the child be able to come home for visits? Some inpatient facilities involve the parents very actively in the child's treatment; others totally exclude the parents. Parents will need to know how they will be treated before allowing the child to enter the facility as an inpatient. In general, it should be noted that if the child will return to live with the parents after inpatient treatment, it is frequently helpful for the parents to be involved in some sort of treatment program while the child is in the facility.

Finally, parents will want to know what procedures will be utilized to evaluate the child's progress in the inpatient facility and what procedures will be utilized to evaluate the child's progress upon return to the home and/or community. There is some evidence that inpatient care (for adolescents, at least) does lead to improvement but that this improvement declines rapidly after the teenagers leave the inpatient facility. Thus, adequate inpatient care involves evaluating the child's progress in the inpatient treatment program, reintegrating the child into the community and/or family, and evaluating the child's progress after returning to the community and/or family. The presumed goal of short-term inpatient treatment is functioning in a community/family, and this goal can be reached only if the child's progress is evaluated both inside and outside the inpatient facility. In some cases, for, example, it will be necessary for the child who leaves the inpatient facility to be engaged in outpatient care to assist in the transition back to the "real world." Inpatient facilities that do not provide assistance in reintegrating the child into the home and/or community are providing less-than-adequate care, and the parent should consider other facilities.

Inpatient treatment is generally only recommended for children who are having very severe difficulties. If such treatment is a step that can be considered well in advance, then the parent can discuss with the professional all the questions indicated above prior to the child's entering the facility. If, on the other hand, inpatient treatment is a response to an emergency situation (for example, the child's having attempted suicide), the parent certainly will not have time to consider all the above questions. In emergency cases, the parent is well advised to have the child hospitalized immediately, and then, if continued inpatient treatment is recommended, to discuss at that time the above questions.

An additional aspect of inpatient treatment should be emphasized. As noted in Chapter 6, inpatient facilities are far more likely than outpatient settings to utilize physical treatments such as medication, electroconvulsive therapy, and psychosurgery. In order to safeguard the child against misuse of these physical treatments, parents need to be careful about what they sign when the child enters the facility. In general, parents should not sign any form permitting the facility to perform any type of physical treatment until after they have discussed the physical treatment with the relevant professional and have evaluated the recommended physical treatment themselves.

Having issued this general caution, it must also be noted that emergency situations can arise where the parent needs to give permission for a medication to be utilized without having evaluated this medication with the professional. Furthermore, some inpatient facilities require parents to give general permission for the use of medication. In such instances, parents can request that some arrangement be made such that the professional has permission to utilize medication as required, but that the professional be committed to informing parents about the use of medication (including the type of medication used and the reason for its use) as soon as possible. Such an arrangement would be designed to give the professional needed treatment flexibility and to give the parents adequate information about the care that their child is receiving.

While parents will sometimes have to give emergency or general permission for the use of medication, *emergency or general permission for electroconvulsive treatment (ECT) or psychosurgery should never be given.* The parent should always carefully evaluate these procedures prior to giving permission for their use. For example, if a hospital requires that parents sign a permission form for ECT prior to admission of the child, the parents will want to carefully consider ECT as a treatment for their child. If the parents decide that ECT is not a good treatment recommendation, then they should refuse to sign the permission form and, because such a hospital usually will not admit the child in the absence of a permission form, take their child elsewhere. As the section below on ECT will indicate, the use of ECT with children is such a questionable procedure that any hospital that requires routine permission to perform ECT on children must be considered a highly questionable treatment facility. The use of psychosurgery with children is an even more dubious and dangerous treatment, as will be discussed below.

Permanent Residence

Placing a child in a mental health facility for permanent residence has typically been called "institutionalizing" a child. Such placements have occurred most frequently for severely mentally retarded children, but sometimes for psychotic children or overly aggressive children as well. Indeed, a generation ago it was not that uncommon for children to be "dumped" into institutions by parents who did not want them, even though the children had no disability that would have merited institutionalization. Fortunately, now this "dumping" has become virtually impossible. Institutions are much more careful about the children they admit, and children must meet certain standards of disability before they will be considered for institutionalization. It should be noted, however, that "dumping" is only one extreme misuse of permanent inpatient care. The other extreme is for parents to keep a severely disabled child at home at a tremendous cost to themselves and to the other children in the family. If maintaining such a child in the home wreaks significant damage on the well-being of other members of the home, the possibility of institutionalizing the child should be seriously considered by the family.

The first step in such a consideration is obtaining an accurate prediction of the child's future development. What is the highest level of functioning that can be reasonably expected of the child? While it is probably impossible for any professional to give an exact answer to this question, it should be possible for a professional, after a very careful evaluation, to give a reasonable estimate. Parents need to know if there is any possibility that the child will ever be able to function independently (or, perhaps, quasi-independently, such as doing tasks around the house or working in a sheltered workshop).

A helpful factor in answering this question is that for most parents the question of institutionalizing the child does not arise until the child has lived at home for several years. Thus, the professional is making a prediction for a child who is, for example, five years old or older. With children this old, it becomes more possible to make more accurate predictive statements. Having even those children with very severe difficulties live in the home for the first few years is a fairly recent development, promoted by the increasing selectivity of institutions and their refusal to admit very young children and by increasing community supports (such as community mental health clinics and special preschool classes) to help the parents maintain the child in the home.

The parent who has obtained a predictive statement from a respected and experienced professional after a careful evaluation is in a position to make a decision about institutionalization. This doesn't mean the decision will be easy: it will typically be very difficult. But at least the parent has the needed information. If the parent feels any doubt about the professional's evaluation procedures and/or predictive statement, a second opinion should be obtained. Only when family members have confidence in the predictive statement offered by the professional will they be able to consider other important factors.

In making a decision about permanent institutionalization, the parent must weigh several factors:

1. The predictive statement (called a "prognosis").
2. The effect of institutionalization on the child.
3. The effect of keeping the child at home on the family.

In considering factors 2 and 3 the following comments may be helpful. First it has to be faced that the effect of institutionalizing most children is more harmful to their social and intellectual development than keeping them in the home would be.[6] This harm is reduced if the child can be placed in an excellent (and typically very expensive) institution. This harm is increased if only custodial care is available at an institution. However, the difference between institutional and home care is less important if the child is profoundly disabled and thus less affected by any environment. The

---

[6] This statement does not necessarily apply to institutions for children with specific disabilities, such as schools for the blind or the deaf, where specific and very important skills are taught to the children in residence, skills they might not be able to learn elsewhere. These types of schools too, however, are beginning increasingly to promote children's maintaining contact with their homes.

benefits of home care are also reduced considerably if the home environment is one of tension and emotional stress as a result of caring for the disabled child.

Factor 3 emphasizes that the effect of the child on other family members must be taken into account. Some families can manage to have the most severely handicapped child in the home, and benefit the child and the rest of the family. Other families simply cannot manage to take care of such a child and still provide a beneficial environment for the rest of the family. After some experience in working with severely disabled children, it is my opinion that it is misleading to consider the first type of family "normal" and the second type "deficient." It is very difficult to maintain a severely disabled child in the home, and I regard those families who can do it well with considerable admiration. Those families who have more difficulties may, in fact, be more "normal"—in the sense of "typical"; it may be that most of us would have difficulty maintaining such a child and benefiting the rest of the family simultaneously.

Taking these three factors into consideration, we can arrive at some rough guidelines. If the prognosis is poor (the child is very unlikely ever to be able to function at any sort of independent level) and if the effect of keeping the child at home is clearly harmful to other members of the family, then I would recommend serious consideration of institutionalizing the child even if the effect on the child will be negative. I would recommend this because the potential harm to others (the other family members) outweighs the potential benefit to the child (since the child has a very limited developmental potential).

On the other hand, if the prognosis is good and the family functions well with the child, then institutionalization is not to be advised. The potential benefit to the child for staying at home is great and the potential harm to others is small.

There are also what we might call mixed cases. If the prognosis is good but the family is having difficulties, I would recommend that family members avail themselves of community supports and attempt to keep the child in the home. Perhaps some sort of day-care setting can be found so that the burdens of caring for the child are eased, but the child maintains his or her place in the home and the community. If the prognosis is poor but the family is having no major difficulties, then the decision is completely up to the family, and most families under these circumstances do decide to keep the child in the home. They have worked out a healthy relationship with the child and they feel no particular desire to institutionalize the child.

Sometimes the prognosis itself is mixed; that is, the professional feels the child has some possibility for independent functioning, but is uncertain how much of a possibility this is. In these cases, I would recommend that one err in favor of the child and treat the prognosis as though it were a good one, thus usually not institutionalizing the child.

Regardless of the original prognostic statement and regardless of the parents' decision about institutionalization, parents should make sure that their child is reevaluated at regular intervals. If a child is institutionalized but later shows more improvement than was expected, most families would want to reconsider their initial decision and think about taking the child back into the home. If, on the other hand, a child who lives at home becomes less able to function and begins to require more care from the rest of the family, the family may have to reconsider the possibility of institutionalization.

While the above guidelines are offered in an attempt to be helpful to families making the decision about institutionalizing their child, it must be stressed that every family must make its own decision. It is hoped that this decision will emphasize the above three factors; but in the final analysis, the family must make the decision with which it is most comfortable. For instance, there may be families who prefer the considerable tension and strain that can be involved in keeping a severely disabled child at home to the guilt and anxiety they would feel if they institutionalized the child. This might not be the decision that I would make, but it may be the best decision for such families. Furthermore, it should be stressed that the entire family should make the decision. This includes the parents, but it also includes the other children in the family, who more than anyone else may feel the effects of having a severely disabled sibling and a tense, overburdened parent.

The family that confronts such a decision will need both information and emotional support. They should avail themselves of discussions with mental health professionals and with any other people in the community who may be of assistance (such as other parents of severely disabled children, physicians, and religious leaders). But after all the advice and consultation are in, the family must make its own decision.

Psychological Treatments That May Be Offered During Inpatient Treatment

Psychological treatments that may be offered during inpatient treatment are the same as those offered on an outpatient basis (for example, psychotherapy, behavior therapy, education) and should be evaluated in the same way. See previous discussions.

Physical Treatments That May Be Offered During Inpatient Treatment

MEDICATION

Medication should be evaluated in an inpatient facility in the same way it would be evaluated when administered to a child living at home. See previous discussion.

ELECTROCONVULSIVE THERAPY

It is difficult for people to be objective about electroconvulsive therapy (ECT). The notion of having electricity passed through one's brain so as to induce a convulsion is so terrifying to most people that it makes it difficult for them to objectively assess its possible therapeutic benefits. This section will try to present the objective facts about ECT to parents, although the conclusion to be drawn may be similar to the one that parents would draw from their emotional reaction. There is, however, an important difference. If parents draw emotional conclusions, they may be rather easily influenced by some authoritative statement by an authoritative person; when parents have read and thought about a more objective consideration, they will be able to make a firmer decision, one that they will be better able to stand by.

Electroconvulsive therapy was originally prescribed for schizophrenic patients because it was thought that epilepsy and schizophrenia rarely occurred together, and thus that the convulsions typical of epilepsy were somehow antagonistic to schizophrenia — that is, if a person had one, he or she could not have the other. As it turned out, both the thought and the treatment were wrong. More careful observation showed that there was no antagonistic relationship between epilepsy and schizophrenia, and ECT proved to be ineffective with schizophrenics (especially as compared to the much greater effectiveness of major tranquilizers such as the phenothiazines). While all of this confusion about ECT and schizophrenia was going on, it was found that ECT did have an impressive beneficial effect on some adults who were deeply depressed. Additionally, some psychotic children were treated with ECT, but this never became a popular form of treatment, and there is no compelling evidence that ECT is an effective treatment for psychotic children.

At present, then, we know the following about ECT:

1. There is no widely accepted evidence that ECT is an effective treatment for schizophrenics of any age.
2. There is no widely accepted evidence that ECT is an effective treatment for psychotic children.
3. There is widely accepted evidence that ECT benefits some adults who are deeply depressed. Since depression in young children is notoriously difficult to identify and may be very different from depression as it is commonly found in adults, this last finding has no implication for the treatment of young children.

Thus, at this time, there is no good scientific basis for administering ECT to any young child. Personally, I would also argue that there is no good scientific basis for administering ECT to most adolescents, although as the adolescent gets older and becomes more adult, ECT might be reasonably considered for a severe, obviously adultlike, depression.

If a professional recommends ECT for a child or adolescent, parents must evaluate this recommendation very carefully. First, no such recommendation should be made unless other treatments (for example, behavior therapy, psychotherapy, medication) have already been tried and have clearly failed. Secondly, I would personally advise that parents always obtain a second opinion and that they make sure that the second opinion comes from a professional who is not personally or professionally associated with the professional who made the initial recommendation. Finally, if both professionals recommend ECT, then parents should ask them for references in the scientific literature that support the use of ECT with children who are similar in age and psychological difficulty to their own child. If parents do not feel comfortable reading this scientific literature by themselves, they can try to find a friend who has had research training to help them, or they can arrange to talk with a mental health professional who has had research training (such as a psychologist at a university or college or a psychiatrist at a medical center).

It should be noted that some mental health professionals would not agree with the caution that I urge in regard to ECT. For this other side, parents might read the writings of Lauretta Bender, a psychiatrist who has utilized ECT with very young children.[7] Views will differ, but I believe that exercising caution can never be a mistake when a physical treatment such

[7] Lauretta Bender, "The Development of a Schizophrenic Child Treated with Electric Convulsions at Three Years of Age" and "Twenty Years of Clinical Research on Schizophrenic Children with Special Reference to Those Under Six Years of Age," in *Emotional Problems of Early Childhood*, edited by Gerald Caplan (New York: Basic Books, 1955), pp. 407-30, 503-18.

as ECT is concerned. In my opinion, parents should only agree to having their child receive ECT when (1) other treatments have been tried and have failed, (2) more than one mental health professional supports this treatment recommendation, and (3) there is clear scientific evidence indicating the effectiveness of ECT for children similar in age and difficulty to the child for whom ECT is being recommended.

PSYCHOSURGERY

Psychosurgery was once a popular treatment for a variety of mental health problems (such as schizophrenia, depression, and excessive anxiety). It was argued that by cutting certain "affective connections" in the brain, people with these mental health problems would be able to respond more normally to their environments. However, when tranquilizing drugs began to be widely used in the 1950s, it was found that, for most people, the drugs were more effective than psychosurgery. Additionally, while the tranquilizers all involved some side effects, their side effects were much milder than the potentially disastrous side effects of any surgical procedure on the brain. Today, psychosurgery is a rarely used treatment. Its use is typically restricted to patients with incurable pain or with mental health problems that have not responded to either psychological treatments or to other physical treatments such as numerous ECT treatments and prolonged drug therapy. While the use of psychosurgery for incurable pain (especially with terminally ill patients) can be a legitimate and humane treatment alternative, some professionals, including myself, question the use of psychosurgery as a treatment for mental health problems. I personally do not believe that we know enough about the relationship between the brain and behavior to offer acceptable chances of obtaining desired behavioral effects through surgical procedures.

Regardless of how professionals stand on the general issue of psychosurgery, they are virtually unanimous in their concern about the use of psychosurgery with children. For example, a recent report on psychosurgery by the National Commission for Protection of Human Subjects of Biomedical and Behavioral Research recommended that children for whom psychosurgery has been recommended be represented by their own lawyer and have a court determine whether or not the treatment recommendation should be carried out. This recommendation of full-scale legal protection for children in regard to psychosurgery indicates the very serious nature of using psychosurgery as a treatment for children.

Thus, if a professional recommends psychosurgery for a child, parents should not consider this a legitimate recommendation unless a variety of other psychological and physical treatments have been tried and have failed. If this is the case, then parents should still be extremely cautious about accepting psychosurgery as a treatment for their child or adolescent. They should obtain a second, independent treatment recommendation. If the second professional supports the recommendation for psychosurgery, then the parents will want to have the professionals involved document their recommendation by referring the parents to the relevant scientific literature. The parents can then consult with someone trained in research methodology to discuss the merits of the research that was conducted. Furthermore, parents will want to consult a lawyer to determine if a court hearing is required and, if it is not required, whether it would be possible to obtain a ourt hearing. This latter procedure might be helpful because the hearing would require that the evidence for and against psychosurgery be presented to the court—and thus to the parents present in court. All of this would be, of course, terribly time-consuming and probably expensive. Consulting organizations such as legal aid societies and community mental health clinics may help to reduce the expense, but the expenditure of time and effort is inevitable. This cost, however, is not too high to pay in evaluating this most extreme and irrevocable treatment.

TREATMENT RECOMMENDATION:
SUPPLEMENTARY TREATMENTS

It has been noted that in providing the best possible mental health care for a child, supplementary treatments (that is, those not directly affecting the child's psychological status, but having important indirect effects) may often be recommended. Examples of such supplementary treatments include speech therapy, physical therapy, dental care, and dietary programs. In evaluating these supplementary treatments, the parents should follow the general guidelines that have been presented throughout this chapter. To illustrate these guidelines as they apply to supplementary treatments, an example is given involving a female adolescent who is overweight in addition to having problems in learning and getting along with her peers.

Guideline	Example
1. The parents should agree with the professional that the child has a specific problem.	In consultation with a physician, the nutritionist states that Joan is overweight but that there is no evidence of a physical problem causing her excessive weight gain.
2. The parents should understand how the supplementary treatment being offered will help the child with this problem. They should also understand how this supplementary treatment will contribute to the child's overall psychological welfare.	A dietary program is offered to Joan and her family. It is believed that this program will help Joan lose weight, while ensuring adequate nutrition. It is also believed that if Joan can lose weight, she will feel better about herself. This may or may not help her improve her learning in school; it should help improve her relationships with her peers.
3. The parents should inquire about any possible harmful effects of the treatment.	Sticking to a diet is hard work, and it may increase tension in the home. The parents will have to modify their behavior with regard to the foods they buy, cook, and eat.
4. The parents should assess the benefit-harm ratio.	After careful consideration, the parents decide that they are willing to run the risk of increased tension in the home and willing to change their own food-related habits in the effort to help Joan stick to her diet. They are willing to do this because they regard Joan's losing weight as very important for her self-confidence and relationships with others.
5. The parents should understand the evaluation procedures to be utilized by the professional who will conduct the supplementary treatment.	The nutritionist will meet with Joan weekly and the family once every two weeks to discuss the diet. Joan will be weighed every week in the clinic. The nutritionist suggests that Joan and her family give the diet a four-month trial period. If at the end of this time Joan has not lost an appropriate amount of weight (around 25 pounds in the nutritionist's opinion), a different approach to weight loss will need to be tried.

Only when parents are satisfied about all five factors should they agree to have the child engage in the recommended supplementary treatment.

> She had quite forgotten the Duchess by this time,
> and was a little startled when she heard her voice close
> to her ear. "You're thinking about something, my dear,
> and that makes you forget to talk. I can't tell you just now
> what the moral of that is, but I shall remember it in a bit."
>
> *Alice's Adventures in Wonderland*

How Do I Discuss Evaluation and Treatment with My Child?

CHAPTER 8

For some parents, the most difficult part about seeking help from a mental health professional is the consultation itself, during which they talk about their concerns and worries with a professional who is initially a stranger to them. Throughout this book, parents have been urged not to let their discomfort about the consultation process stand in the way of their obtaining professional advice when they feel they and their child need it.

For other parents, while the consultation process may be somewhat uncomfortable, at least at first, their major discomfort comes when they have to explain the consultation process to their child. This need to explain begins with the child's first contact with the professional, which is, as noted in Chapter 5, usually concerned with obtaining an evaluation of the child's psychological functioning. The need for explanation, however, doesn't stop here. After the evaluation, the child needs to understand the results of the evaluation, and if treatment is recommended, he or she needs to understand the nature of that process as well. Many, many parents feel awkward and anxious about when and how they are to discuss these issues with their child. This chapter is presented as a source of some general advice that, hopefully, will reduce some of these feelings of discomfort and allow for more beneficial communication between parent and child.

EXPLAINING WHY THE FAMILY IS GOING TO A MENTAL HEALTH FACILITY

If the child is very young — say, under two years of age — or has great difficulty understanding verbal communications, it is essentially impossible to give him or her detailed reasons about going to a mental health facility. A positive attitude by the parent is probably the most important factor, accompanied by some positive, simple statement such as "We're going to see some nice people who will like you." More complicated explanations indicating parental concern about, for example, mental retardation or psychosis are out of place with very young or severely language-impaired children, and may serve to convey anxiety rather than reassurance.

If, however, the child is able to understand verbal communication, a more detailed discussion is necessary. Parents do not suddenly take their children to mental health facilities. First of all they become worried about the child, and then they consult a facility. In the majority of cases, the parents' first response to their concern will be, and should be, to talk it over with the child. In this talk, parents should be careful not to accuse the child of anything, but should instead state their concerns. For example:

- I'm worried about your grades in school.
- or
- I'm worried about your wetting the bed.
- or
- I'm worried about how you seem to me to be feeling sad a lot.
- or
- I'm worried about whether you're taking drugs.
- or
- I'm worried about your sexual behavior.

Whatever the worry is, it should be stated to the child in direct, simple terms that are truthful and that the child can understand. Many times, the discussion that will ensue will provide all that is needed to correct the problem. Parents may find out that their worry is unfounded, or the child may be able to explain what is causing the problem and together with the parent work to change things so as to reduce the problem. Sometimes, however, the discussion will indicate that a problem does in fact exist, but parent and child will be unable to come up with a solution for it. Other times, the child will say the problem doesn't exist, but the parent continues to believe it does. Let us take these last examples one by one to indicate how parents can respond.

1. Discussion indicates a problem exists, but a solution can't be found. This is probably the easiest situation in terms of what happens next. Parents may begin to think that if they and the child can't solve the problem, they need some outside help. The parent can suggest this to the child, talk it out with the child, and, in most cases, come to an agreement that some outside help will be sought. In this case, going to a mental health facility is readily understandable to the child; he or she has helped come to the decision to go. Children in these circumstances still need to be told what exactly will happen there, but at least they know why they are going.

1a. The solution arrived at by parent and child doesn't work. In this case, the parent needs to discuss with the child the solution that was tried and why it failed. In this discussion, parent and child may come to feel that they need outside help in devising a better solution. Once this is felt, then this situation is identical to the one described above (1).

2. Child says problem doesn't exist, or when obtaining outside help is suggested by the parent (as in 1 and 1a above), the child doesn't agree. In these situations, the child will not be a willing participant in going to a mental health facility. The parent who is responsible for the child's welfare must take this responsibility in hand and consult the facility even if the child doesn't want to. To help avoid conflict between parent and child over this, this course of action can be explained to the child along the following lines:

"I know you think that I'm worrying needlessly [or: that we don't need to bring anyone else in on this], but I am still worried. I feel strongly that we need to see a mental health professional about this. This person will be able to be objective about the situation, listen to each of us, and help us arrive at some reasonable solution. If I'm worrying needlessly, then this is what I will be told and then I will stop bugging you. But I'm just never going to be sure unless we see someone about this. You don't have to *want* to go, all I'm asking you to do is to *go* and to explain your view of things."

This sort of explanation places the responsibility for going on the parent and not on the presumed problem of the child. Thus, going to the professional does not entail forcing the child to admit to having a problem. All that is acknowledged by going is that the parent thinks the child has a problem and that the parent is therefore worried. The professional can be viewed in this case as a referee, an arbitrator, someone who will hear conflicting points of view and attempt to come up with some reasonably satisfactory answer for all parties. Because of their professional training and their lack of emotional involvement with either the parents or the child, mental health professionals are in a position to do this. It is very important that both parents and child in this situation realize the objective position of the professional, and that neither view the professional as an ally against the other. The professional will try to act in the best interests of both the parents and child.

All these discussions have to be put in terms that the child can comprehend, but this should be possible for all parents and children except where the child is so young or has such severe problems of understanding verbal communication that this is not feasible. Except for these children, all other children who arrive at a mental health facility should know fairly precisely why they are there (for example: I wet my bed and mom and dad are worried about it). Children who are thus informed are equipped to make the most efficient use of their contacts with the mental health facility and are spared unnecessary anxiety and confusion.

EXPLAINING WHAT WILL HAPPEN AT A MENTAL HEALTH FACILITY

In addition to understanding why they are there, children who are brought to a mental health facility should understand what will happen to them at the facility. All too often, I have seen children brought to a mental health facility who have been told by their parents they are going to see "the doctor." Now if a psychiatrist (who is a physician, as explained earlier, p. 51 will be involved, this way of informing the child does have a certain truth to it, but the overall effect of the communication may still be misleading. Many children fear "the doctor," who represents to them that person who does unpleasant things to them such as pushing a "stick" down their throat or giving them a shot. Consequently, mental health professionals frequently have to explain to children that they are not that kind of doctor, and that they will not give them a shot or any kind of physical examination at all. There is really no need for mental health professionals to have to explain this; the child could have been told this prior to coming to the facility, saving a lot of confusion and as least some of the anxiety. Thus, it is very important for parents to begin making truthful and important distinctions for the child from the very first contact with the mental health facility.

The best way to begin is for parents themselves to understand exactly what will happen during the child's first visit. If the facility wishes to see the child during the first visit, the parent can inquire over the phone about what experiences the child will have. If the facility wishes to see the parent on the first visit and the child on a later one, the parent can inquire prior to the child's visit what experiences the child will have. Knowing what will happen, the parent should communicate this clearly to the child.

Often, for instance, the only thing that happens during a first visit is that someone talks with the child. The parent should explain this in some manner similar to the following example:

"We are going to the child guidance clinic. They work with many children there to help the children feel better about themselves and get along better [in school, with others — whatever fits the specific child]. Someone there will'talk with you about how you feel about things. That's all that will happen. The clinic is *not* like the doctor's or the dentist's. No one there will give you a shot or work with your teeth. They will only talk with you."

This kind of explanation should be given in terms that the child can understand and should be appropriate to his or her age and language skills. Having received such an explanation, children will have a good idea of what to expect and shouldn't have to worry about what will happen to them.

We should note that in some settings that deal with both emotional and physical problems — a developmental evaluation clinic, for example — the first visit does sometimes involve a physical examination. If a physical is to be given, this should be explained to the child. In this case, saying the child will see "a doctor" is appropriate and correct. If, however, other things are to happen such as people talking with the child or a psychologist administering tests, these too should be explained to the child beforehand.

In terms of a psychologist seeing a child for evaluation purposes, it might be helpful for me to indicate what I tell a child before a psychological evaluation. If the child is quite young (six or under), I typically say something along the following lines: "I'm going to play some games with you, talk with you, and ask you some questions. I have some toys that I think you'll like." Since most psychological tests for young children are designed to interest them and involve materials that do in fact resemble toys, this explanation serves very well to prepare such children for what they will do. If the child is older, I usually say something like: "I'm a psychologist and I'm interested in what you feel and think about things. I will want to talk with you about your feelings and thoughts. I will also want you to work on some materials I have so that I can find out what things you're good at and what things are more difficult for you." These kinds of explanations can be given by the parent prior to the child's coming to the facility and, if given, would be a great help in getting the child's visit off to a good start.

It should be noted here that if parents wish to describe to the child what will happen, but believe that they don't know enough to do so, they should feel free to talk with the professional about this issue. For instance, if a psychological evaluation is scheduled, but parents feel they don't quite know how to describe this to the child, the parents should talk with the psychologist about this. The psychologist would then explain to the parents what will happen and work out with the parents a good way to describe this to the child. If any professional indicates that he or she does not think it is part of their job to help the parent prepare the child for the child's visit, then the parent may wish to go to someone else who more clearly recognizes the child's need for preparation.

Once the initial visit is over, it will generally be easier to prepare the child for future visits. The child will be familiar now with the facility and with at least some of the people in it. The child will have found out, for instance, that no shots are given; indeed, many children enjoy the attention they receive. The parent should, however, keep in close consultation with the professional directing the child's evaluation experiences. Anytime a new and different evaluation procedure is about to occur, the parent should prepare the child for this. Through careful preparation, children will be better able to trust the clinic and will feel secure that their parents are helping them through the experience rather than hiding something from them.

AFTER THE EVALUATION

When an evaluation of a child is concluded, it is customary procedure for the professional to meet with the parents to discuss the findings of the evaluation. Usually some sort of feedback session will also be arranged for the child. There are many different methods of scheduling such sessions depending on the specific child and problem and family situation. For example, the professional may meet with parents and child together for all feedback sessions. Or the professional may meet with the parents alone, then the child alone, and then the parents and child together. While the exact scheduling of sessions should be left to the professional's discretion, parents usually should expect that the child will receive some feedback from the professional and that at least one session will be held involving both parents and child.

During a feedback session, there are two major concerns. First, there is the professional's evaluation of the nature of the child's problem. Secondly, there are treatment recommendations. Both of these are major issues to the child as well as to the parents. Children who come to mental health facilities are frequently quite anxious that "something's wrong with me." Good preparation—stating the reason for coming to the facility in clear, nonaccusatory language—can diminish this concern, but some concern will almost inevitably persist. Thus, if parents and professionals were not to tell the child about the results of the evaluation, such a child might well assume the worst—that something is indeed "wrong" and that it's so bad no one wants to talk about it. To prevent the child from reaching such a conclusion, it is very important to tell the child in clear, nonaccusatory language what the professional thinks is the problem of concern and what is being recommended to help with the problem. If they meet the professional alone, without the child, the parents can discuss with the professional how to convey this information to the child. Perhaps best of all, however, the parents can observe the way the professional conveys this information during a joint session. They can learn, through observing, the best way to tell the child so as to be sure he or she understands and so as to reduce anxiety.

In order to give parents an idea of how psychological problems and their treatment can be explained, the following examples are offered. These examples are general ones and will not apply to all children with each type of problem that is considered. Talking to children about the nature of their difficulties must be tailored to the age, level of sophistication, and emotional stability of the individual child. In spite of these important qualifications, however, it may be helpful for many parents to read some examples of how professionals go about explaining the result of an evaluation to children with a variety of mental health problems. Having read such examples, parents should be in a better position to talk with or observe a professional and learn how to explain the results of an evaluation to their own child.

EXAMPLES OF DISCUSSING
MENTAL HEALTH PROBLEMS WITH CHILDREN

Mental Retardation

Cindy, as you know, we've given you a lot of things to do since you started coming to the clinic. We asked you a lot of questions, we had you work with some materials. . . . Remember trying to put the picture puzzles together? Now, all of this was done so we could get some idea of what things were easy for you and what things were difficult for you. You remember that one of the reasons you came to us with your mom and dad was that you were having trouble in school. After working with you during this time we have found that the reason you have trouble in school is because you have more trouble learning than a lot of your classmates. This doesn't mean that you're lazy or don't try—we know that you try very hard. It does mean that something like spelling will be more difficult for you than for many of your classmates.

Have you ever heard the words *mental retardation?* What do you think they mean? [Give the child a chance to answer; typical answers include "it means people who are dumb."] Well, then, what does "dumb" mean? ["It means people who are stupid, who can't do things."] Does dumb mean that the person is bad? ["No."] Does it mean that the person can't do *anything*—like play ball, or help mother out around the house, or be a good friend? ["No."] Okay, let me tell you what mental retardation means to me. It means that some people have more trouble with thinking out problems than others. So school is going to be harder for them, and sometimes things like getting change at the store will be harder. But it doesn't mean they can't do anything, or that they're bad people, or that they can't learn. I think you're a very good person and I know there are many things you can do. And I know you can learn. In order to help you learn more, I want to help you and your parents arrange for some special teaching . . . [specific treatment recommendations would be given here].

Learning Disability

Tom, as you know, we've given you a lot of things to do since you started coming to the clinic. We asked you a lot of questions, we had you work with some materials. . . . Remember trying to put the picture puzzles together? Now, all of this was done so we could get some idea of what things were easy for you and what things were difficult for you. You remember that one of the reasons you came to us with your dad was that you were having trouble in school. Now after working with you during this time, we have found out two important things. One thing we have found out is that you are behind in your school subjects. You have trouble reading, some trouble with spelling, and lots of trouble with math. Another thing we've learned, however, is that your ability to learn is normal. Now it's very important for you to think about both of these things. You are behind in school, but you do have normal ability to learn.

Do you know what *mental retardation* means? ["Dumb."] Do you think you're mentally retarded? ["Some kids at school called me retardo."] Well, I want you to know that you're not mentally retarded. To be mentally retarded means that a person has lots of trouble with all kinds of learning. You only have trouble with specific kinds of learning: the kind you're expected to do in school. I know from talking with you that you can learn quite a bit under certain circumstances: like about "Star Trek," for example. You are not dumb; you do have trouble learning certain things in school. Now one of the questions you may think of, right now or later when you think it over, is how you could be normal in learning *ability*, but have trouble learning in school. To tell you the truth, I just don't know the answer to that. I know it is not because you're lazy or not trying. I saw you try very hard on that reading test but you still could not do it. It may be that you could learn more if you were taught a different way. For that reason, I want to recommend to you and your dad . . . [specific treatment recommendation would be given here].

Enuresis (Bed Wetting)

You remember, Frank, that when you came here, you and your mom were concerned because you were wetting the bed. One of the things that we here at the clinic wanted to find out was whether there was any physical problem that was making you wet your bed. Remember how we had you go see Dr. Jones? Well, Dr. Jones has told us that you're perfectly healthy physically, so that's not the reason. Another thing we want to know about was how you and your mom got along. Sometimes boys and girls wet their beds when they're mad at their parents or feel they're not getting enough attention. Remember how we talked with both of you about that, and had mom keep count of how much time the two of you spent together. Well, it looks to us as if you're pretty happy at home, get a lot of attention, and aren't mad at your mom. So, we think that you may be wetting your bed because, for some reason, you never learned to wake up in time at night to make it to the toilet. So we're going to try installing an alarm system in your bed at night. Let me tell you how this system will work . . . [specifics of treatment recommendation given here].

Emotional Difficulties within the Family

Elizabeth, remember how when you came here to the clinic, both you and your mom were worried about your not going to school, yelling so much at home, and throwing things at people? Your dad didn't feel there was much of a problem, but as we've found out when we've talked together, your dad doesn't spend much time at home. Now we've had you and your parents do a lot of things here: we've talked to the three of you, alone and together; we've had each of you count how much time the three of you spend together; we've had you count when you yell and throw things. After all of this, we've come to the conclusion that you're acting the way you are, *not* because something is "wrong with you," but because you're upset about the way things are going at home. We know that you get very upset when your mom and dad fight, and we know that they've been fighting a lot lately. We also know that you don't understand why they're fighting. We think that the only way to make you feel better and help you to control yourself better is to talk over things with the whole family. This way of working with an entire family is called "family therapy." What it involves is . . . [specifics of treatment recommendation given here].

It is important to note that no matter how well done, the feedback given to the child by the professional is just the beginning. The parents will need to make sure the child understands the feedback, and this may involve additional sessions with the professional and will certainly involve discussion of the feedback among the parents and child when they are at home.

Children also need to understand whatever treatment is recommended. In each of the examples above, the professional statement left off at the point at which the treatment recommendation would be given and described. It will usually be the case that a statement of the problem will lead naturally into a statement of the recommended treatment. It is very important that children understand what experiences are being recommended for them. They should discuss how they feel about the recommendation and should raise any objections they have to it with their parents and the professional. If the treatment recommendations are followed, the child who is well informed will be much less anxious about what is to happen and will be able to benefit more from the treatment procedures.

Thus in working with children, a paramount concern is to keep them informed about what is happening during their contact with the clinic. They need to be prepared ahead of evaluation and treatment, and they need to be informed along the way about any changes or conclusions. With very young children or children whose ability to understand verbal communications is very limited, this explanation procedure is necessarily more limited. For these children, as noted, parental attitude is probably the most important element. For more verbally skilled children, however, more information must be provided. This information when presented properly and tailored to the individual child will make a strong contribution to a successfull consultation with a mental health facility.

THE ROLE OF OTHER FAMILY MEMBERS

So far in describing how parents might go about discussing mental health evaluation and treatment with their child, issues have been presented as though only the parents and the child were involved. In many families, of course, there are other family members who will be aware that there is some sort of difficulty and who may be aware that a mental health facility is being consulted. These other family members include most often brothers and/or sisters of the child, but others, such as grandparents or uncles and aunts, may also be involved. Additionally, there are many divorced couples with children, and the family situation after a divorce may include a stepfather and/or stepmother in addition to the child's biological parents.

While individual parents will have to work out for themselves exactly how much they wish other family members to know about their consultation of a mental health facility, some general guidelines may prove useful. Essentially, there are two major issues to keep in mind. The first is that for parents not to inform other family members about anything that goes on at the mental health facility runs the risk of creating a web of secrecy that is very confusing and very hard to maintain. It also may indicate to the child that going to the mental health facility is something shameful and that he or she should be ashamed both of going and of the problems that led to going. Secondly, however, the parents should feel firmly that their activities at a mental health facility are confidential and that they have every right to protect their privacy. Thus, these two issues are often in conflict: consideration of the first indicating that other family members should be informed; consideration of the second indicating that other family members should not be informed.

I want to suggest to parents that either of these extreme positions is probably a mistake. Parents who say nothing to other family members may get caught in a web of secrecy. Parents who tell everything to other family members may feel their privacy has been invaded. Most parents will probably want to work out some middle-of-the-road approach, telling other family members enough so that confusion is not created and the child does not feel ashamed about going to the mental health facility, but keeping to themselves any information that would make them uncomfortable for it to become public knowledge.

I would also urge that parents and child talk over together how much and what they are going to tell other family members. During this discussion, both parents and child will have the opportunity to ask that specific information be kept confidential and, by agreeing in advance about how they will talk to other family members, will be able to avoid the unpleasant confusion that can arise from different people saying different things. This prior discussion should not be held in an atmosphere of "Let's get together so we can keep our story straight with grandma," but in an atmosphere of "Going to the community mental health center is very important to all of us, and we may want to keep some things private. How can we best tell grandma what we do there so she will understand, and yet not have to talk about anything we want to keep private?"

A special comment at this point should be made about discussing mental health evaluation and treatment of children with their brothers and/or sisters. As members of the family who live with the parents and the child, these siblings will always know when the parents are worried and when anything unusual, such as going to a mental health facility, is happening. It is absolutely impossible to keep such information from them. If, indeed, an effort is made to keep such information from them, they may well conclude that something quite terrible is going on. Therefore, no matter what one does about other, more distant, family members, it is always important to discuss what is happening at the mental health facility with the child's brothers and/or sisters. Even with siblings, however, parents and the child have a right not to tell them specific information that they wish to keep private.

In many instances a good approach would be for the parents and child to have a family gathering, with all the brothers and sisters present, and discuss something of the nature of the problem and of their evaluation and/or treatment activities at the facility. Presuming the parents and child have discussed this family gathering prior to its occurrence, any information that anyone wants to be kept private can simply not be disclosed at this time. If, as sometimes happens, the siblings persist in making a mysterious or fearful thing out of the family's going to a mental health facility, the parents and child may want to take them to the facility for a visit. Once siblings have seen the facility and met the professional with whom the family is working, they frequently decide it's all pretty boring and not such a big deal after all. This attitude, while it may come as something of a shock to the parents and child who are intensely involved in their consultation with the facility, is a great improvement over the fearful and bewildered fantasies it replaces.

> Better say nothing at all. Language is worth a thousand pounds a word!
>
> Through the Looking-Glass

How Do I Pay for Mental Health Care?

CHAPTER 9

In Chapter 3, there was some brief mention of the different rates and methods of payment for mental health care. The present chapter will offer some more details on these issues, although, as will be seen, only very general statements are possible in the light of extreme variation among professionals, facilities, and insurance companies. The major purposes of this chapter, then, are to give parents some general ideas about the various rates and methods of payment, and to make it clear that for any specific professional, facility, or insurance company, parents will have to check carefully to find out the exact cost of mental health care for their child.

OUTPATIENT FACILITIES

Evaluation

As noted in Chapter 3, the major types of facilities that a parent may take a child to for an evaluation include developmental evaluation clinics, private practitioners, child guidance clinics, community mental health centers, and departments of psychiatry. The evaluation of the child's difficulties that is obtained at any of these facilities will, of course, cost money. The method of charging for such services may be based either on hourly rates (so much per hour per professional) or on a fixed evaluation fee (so much for the typical sorts of evaluation procedures, such as psychological testing, with additional costs for any unusual evaluation procedures). Parents should inquire as to how the price for the evaluation is determined and make sure that they know what price is being charged for what specific service. Regardless of the method of charging, however, parents will then have to consider how to pay for the evaluation. If they do not have insurance, it will be very important to them whether the facility charges on a sliding scale or by a fixed rate. A sliding scale — frequently utilized in, for example, child guidance clinics and community mental health centers — means that costs are set according to parental income (or sometimes in the case of older adolescents, the child's income). Insurance coverage is also usually considered when charges are based on a sliding scale fee system.[1] Thus, the more money parents make (or the more insurance they have), the more they are charged for services, up to a certain limit. This upper limit is usually equivalent to the rate that a facility not using a sliding scale fee system would charge. So even if parents have substantial income and/or insurance coverage, they are not financially disadvantaged by the sliding scale, in that they pay no more than they would if no sliding scale were in effect. For parents whose income and/or insurance coverage is less substantial, the sliding scale system offers significant reductions in cost over a facility that does not utilize a sliding scale fee system. This reduction is most important for parents who are not eligible for governmental assistance programs, do not have insurance, and are, therefore, paying cost directly.

For those parents who have insurance, most insurance companies will cover the cost of an evaluation. Some may cover all of this cost; others may cover only part of the cost. Some may pay only when a psychiatrist (M.D.) has supervised the evaluation; others will pay if any qualified professional (for example, either a psychologist or psychiatrist) has been in charge. Parents should talk with a representative of the insurance company covering them to find out the company's specific policy on paying for evaluations. Evaluations at developmental evaluation clinics are usually especially easy to have covered by insurance companies since much of the evaluation is medical (pediatric) in nature.

[1]Some facilities also consider the number of dependents and/or existing financial obligations that parents have in establishing charges on a sliding scale basis.

Some departments of psychiatry utilize sliding fees and others do not. Private practitioners generally do not utilize sliding scale fees, although a few might. If a facility does not utilize a sliding scale system, then the parent will be charged at the going rate, either an hourly or fixed evaluation fee as noted above. This can typically be quite expensive: $35 to $50 an hour is not unusual as an hourly rate, and $150 to $200 as a fixed evaluation fee is fairly common. For parents directly paying, this represents a substantial investment.

Thus, for an evaluation, the parent should inquire about the following aspects of cost:

1. Is payment based on an hourly rate, or is there a fixed evaluation fee? If the latter, what is being paid for?
2. Does the facility use a sliding scale fee system? If so, how would it apply to me?
3. What is the estimated total cost of the evaluation?
4. Do I have insurance coverage or governmental assistance for this cost? (This must be determined by consulting a representative of the company issuing the policy, or an official of the governmental agency.)

Treatment

There are many similarities and some differences between payment for evaluations and payment for treatment in the types of outpatient facilities we have been discussing. Most payment for treatment is based on an hourly rate (so much per hour per professional). Fixed fee charging is fairly unusual, although one does find it for parental effectiveness training (PET) courses, where a fixed fee is charged for a specified number of PET sessions. As with evaluation, child guidance clinics and community mental health centers frequently utilize a sliding scale fee system for treatment costs. Some departments of psychiatry utilize such a system, while private practitioners rarely utilize a sliding scale system. Again, a sliding scale system can significantly reduce costs, and this is especially important if the parent does not have insurance coverage or governmental assistance.

Hourly rates of $35 to $50 are not uncommon in the absence of a sliding scale fee system, or for parents whose income falls in the upper category of a sliding scale fee system. If treatment is conducted once a week at, for example $35 an hour for one year (minus a four-week vacation), this would amount to $1,680, and is, obviously, a significant financial investment. More frequent treatment sessions, or a longer duration of treatment, or a more expensive hourly rate would, of course, all increase this cost. For a family with a low income and no outside assistance, a sliding scale fee system can reduce the cost to essentially nothing. I have worked in a facility where per-hour cost for very-low-income families amounted to 25 cents, or $12 a year using the example cited above. Obviously, then, parents with a low level of income and without outside assistance will want to determine whether the facility they are considering for treatment utilizes a sliding scale fee system.

For those parents who have insurance, the amount of coverage for mental health treatment available to them under their insurance policy often comes as something of a shock. Many companies pay only a portion of the per-session cost (for example, 50 percent) and will cover only a specified number of sessions. For example, consider a company that will only pay 50 percent of the cost for 25 sessions. Using the above example of a once a week, $35 a session, 48 weeks' duration, this company would pay only $437.50, leaving the parents to pay $1,242.50. Furthermore, some companies have very restrictive rules about whom they will pay for treatment (such as only psychiatrists), while others are more flexible (such as paying for treatment by other mental health professionals as well). Finally, many insurance companies are apparently rather vague about what or whom they will pay in regard to mental health treatment. I have been told by administrative assistants in charge of filing for insurance that they recommend to parents that they always file for insurance payment regardless of what their policy appears to say because, as one put it, "Sometimes the insurance companies will pay and sometimes they won't; you never know until you actually file for payment."

All of this apparent confusion about insurance leads to some guidelines for parents. Certainly, if treatment for one's child has been recommended, parents need to discuss with a representative of their insurance company what the company will cover; they may, in addition, be advised to file regardless of what the agent or the policy states. A little preventive action might, however, be the best approach. I would advise any parent, or prospective parent, to try to ascertain that company with the best coverage of mental health treatment when they are initially considering what policy to purchase. This information can then be a factor when they make their decision about which company to purchase insurance from. Also, parents involved in companies that are contracting for group insurance might urge their employers to find out about these provisions and make this information known to the employees before deciding which company to contract with. The best way to ensure adequate insurance coverage is to purchase insurance that offers the best coverage, always provided, of course, that one can afford the cost of paying for such coverage. It takes a little time and effort to investigate insurance companies policies on mental health coverage, but it is well worth the time and effort if one is ever called upon to utilize this coverage. Putting in this initial time and effort may protect parents from the very considerable shock some have had who thought they were well covered and then, when they needed the coverage, found out they were not.

The summary of the inquiries parents need to make when considering the cost of treatment is slightly different from that which was given for the consideration of evaluation costs:

1. If at all possible and economically feasible, get the best coverage for mental health treatment when you are purchasing insurance, before you actually have need of such coverage.
2. When treatment is recommended, inquire about the following:
    a. Is payment based on an hourly rate? If so, what is that rate?
    b. For hourly rates, what is the professional's estimate of how many hours will be needed? For example, how many hours a week will be scheduled? How many weeks, or months, or years is treatment expected to last?
    c. If payment is not based on an hourly rate, is it based on a fixed fee? If so, what is that fee? What does is include?
    d. For fixed rates, are there additional anticipated costs? What are they? How much will they cost?
    e. Is there a sliding scale? If so, how would it apply to me?
    f. What is the estimated total cost of treatment?
3. Parents who have insurance need to inquire about the following from their insurance agent:
    a. What proportion of the cost of each treatment session is covered?
    b. How many sessions are covered?
    c. What type(s) of professionals are covered?
    d. If coverage appears inadequate: Is there any way to extend coverage?

INPATIENT FACILITIES

Evaluation

Extensive initial evaluation procedures for children in inpatient settings are rather rare. Typically, children are evaluated prior to coming to the inpatient setting. There may be, however, a less extensive evaluation to determine whether or not to admit the child to the facility, and there frequently are periodic evaluations to assess the child's progress during his or her residence in the facility. Evaluation costs in an inpatient setting are usually considered part of the total inpatient costs and as such would be subject to the general principles noted below for inpatient treatment.

Treatment

Essentially there are two kinds of financing categories relevant to mental health services for inpatients: public and private. These categories are reflected in the types of inpatient mental health facilities found in the United States: public (for example, state psychiatric hospitals) and private (for example, privately run psychiatric hospitals). This distinction is made according to how the facility is funded. Public facilities are supported, in large part, by governmental (local, state, and/or federal) funds; private facilities get most of their funds from costs charged to patients. This distinction between government and individual funding also applies to facilities such as general hospitals that are funded by a mixture of public and private sources. Many general hospitals have both "public" and "private" patients; the costs for the public patients are paid by governmental funds, while the costs for the private patients are paid by the patients themselves. The following discussion considers these two types of financing categories, public versus private, in some more detail.

PUBLIC FUNDING

When their child is receiving inpatient treatment at a public institution or is classified as a "public patient" at any type of facility, costs to the parents will vary depending on the facility and the state in which the facility is located. Sometimes, parents will have to contribute financially to the care of their child, and usually such contributions will be based on a sliding scale fee system worked out for the total cost of inpatient care relative to parental income. For parents who have a substantial income, these fees can be quite expensive for some institutions in some states. In other states and other facilities, costs are relatively low regardless of income. In all states and all facilities, costs to very-low-income parents without insurance coverage will be low or nonexistent. When fees are charged for children considered to be public patients, parents can pay either through their insurance coverage or out of pocket. It is important to remember that in determining parents' income for use with a sliding scale fee system, "income" includes not only what the parents earn but also the amount of insurance coverage they carry. Thus, if a parent earns a relatively low income but has good insurance coverage, the parent might be charged (through claims on his or her insurance) a fairly high cost by those facilities that charge for "public" care.

PRIVATE FUNDING

For private institutions, or "private patients" in a general hospital, the cost is usually borne by insurance coverage. It would be theoretically possible for someone to pay this cost out of pocket, but since we are talking about *very* high expenses (such as $50 a day and up), one would have to be quite wealthy to pay for this kind of care without insurance coverage. Additionally, it should be noted that while it is possible for inpatient treatment to be fairly brief (for example, a week), it can be of very long duration (six months to a year not being at all ususual). Sometimes, of course, for those children who are not able to function independently and whose families have made the decision not to keep them at home, inpatient care can last the length of the individual's life.

Determining insurance coverage for inpatient care is generally less confusing than that for outpatient care. There can, however, be some surprises in store for parents. Many insurance companies will pay only a percentage of the inpatient costs (although this tends to be a fairly high percentage, such as 80 percent), and many will cover inpatient care only up to a certain limit. Additionally, many companies will pay only facilities that meet certain criteria, and they may not pay for supplementary treatment (such as educational tutoring). So while almost all insurance companies will pay something for inpatient treatment, and while that sum tends to be a considerable amount, they may not pay as much as is needed to cover the full cost of treatment.

QUESTIONS TO ASK ABOUT INPATIENT TREATMENT

When considering the financial aspects of inpatient treatment, parents need to find answers to the following questions:

1. Is the facility (or patient status) public or private?
2. What is the professional's best estimate of the length of stay and types of treatments that will be necessary?
3. In light of the above factors, what is the best estimate of total cost?
4. What is the maximum amount the insurance company will pay for inpatient treatment? Are there any restrictions placed by the company on

payment (for example, type of facility, type of treatment)? The answer to this question must be determined by consultation with a representative of the insurance company issuing the policy.
5. What is the difference between 3 and 4? Does the parent's insurance cover all costs, or will the parents need to pay for part of the cost? If the parents will need to pay, how much will they need to pay?
   a. If the facility or patient status is public and the parents can easily afford the costs (either through insurance or out of pocket), the parents may want to check on whether they could afford the costs of a private facility or with the child as a private patient.
   b. If the facility or patient status is private and the parents can afford the costs, then they can be comfortable with the financial aspects of the recommended treatment.
   c. If the facility or patient status is public and the parents cannot afford the cost, then they will want to talk with the professional staff at the facility to see if they can obtain a reduction in cost.
   d. If the facility or patient status is private and the parents cannot afford the cost, then they will want to investigate costs for treatment of the child as a public patient or at a public facility.

WHAT DOES IT MEAN, ALL THIS TALK ABOUT MONEY?

Most parents when they take their child to a mental health facility do not think about money. They are concerned about their child, they want help, and money is the furthest thing from their minds. At some point, however, parents have to consider the financial aspect. Often this consideration will be a very complex weighing of the benefits of treatment against the possible problems caused by a large expenditure of money. But before this consideration can even begin, parents need to know how much money they will have to pay. This chapter has been written to help the parent figure out what this sum will be. Parents are urged to ask about expenses—even though it should be recognized that it is hard to give an exact cost statement for what treatment will cost (it's usually easier to be more exact about evaluation costs). Thus, even though the cost estimate parents receive is just that—an estimate—it can still serve as a baseline from which parents can estimate how much they can expect to have to pay.

Payment, of course, is just one of the issues parents will need to consider. Let us take the case of inpatient care to highlight the complexity of the other issues with which payment is involved. Let us suppose that a parent—we can call him Mr. Campbell—discovers that a recommended private facility for his child is likely to cost him some $10,000 a year more than his insurance coverage will provide. This is a great deal of money for most people. In addition, let us suppose that Mr. Campbell is told that a public facility will provide inpatient care for his child at essentially no cost to him. Clearly, on financial grounds, the public facility is the better choice. There are, however, other factors to be considered. Mr. Campbell will want to inquire about the quality of care available in the two facilities, and it may well be that the private facility provides better care than the public one. Thus, on the grounds of the child's welfare, the private facility is the better choice. Now add to this situation the not-uncommon additional factor that Mr. Campbell has other children whose standard of living will be significantly reduced if he has to go into debt in order to pay the costs of the private institution. And furthermore, add the question about how likely it is that any treatment at any facility will result in significant improvement in his child's problems. Consideration of the other children will make Mr. Campbell reluctant to bear the added cost. In the case of a good prognosis (the child is likely to improve), consideration of the child's prognosis, will make Mr. Campbell more willing to bear the cost or, in the case of a poor prognosis (the child is unlikely to improve) less willing to bear the cost.

Parents caught in this kind of dilemma should have help in considering the various possibilities. These parents need to discuss the above issues, and any other ones affecting their decision, with the professional who is recommending the treatment. The professional has an obligation not only to recommend treatment, but to discover with the parents the most reasonable treatment that is available—reasonable in terms of quality, expense, prognosis, and entire family context. Parents are sometimes embarrassed to discuss the financial aspects of treatment with a professional. They feel that they are "bad" parents if they mention cost when treatment for their child is being recommended. Parents should not feel embarrassed at mentioning cost, nor should they feel they're not being good parents when doing so.

Indeed, part of being a good parent to a child with mental health problems is to carefully consider the cost of the recommended treatment. This is important because if parents agree to treatments they cannot afford, they will either have to stop the child's treatment when the cost becomes too high or they will suffer through intolerable financial burdens that at some point will adversely affect their relationship to the child's treatment and, most likely, their relationship to the child. Parents should only agree to treatments that they can afford; agreeing to affordable treatments will mean that parents will be able to wholeheartedly assist and support the treatment and the child. The financial cost of mental health care is a fact. It must be openly discussed and considered by both professionals and parents.

> "Take some more tea," the March Hare said to Alice, very earnestly.
> "I've had nothing yet," Alice replied in an offended tone: "so I can't take more."
> "You mean you can't take *less*," said the Hatter: "it's very easy to take *more* than nothing."
>
> Alice's Adventures in Wonderland

Rights and Responsibilities

CHAPTER 10

This book has emphasized parents' rights to be well informed and to make decisions concerning their child's mental health care. The guiding assumption has been that parents are sensitive to their child's needs and will obtain the best possible care for the child within the context of their specific family situation. I firmly believe that this is most typically the case. Parents come to mental health facilities desiring help for their child. Not uncommonly, they may also need assistance for themselves. They may need to change their expectations with regard to the child, to modify their child-rearing practices, or to examine their own emotional responses to the child. Whatever type of assistance is needed, the vast majority of parents have good intentions and are the best possible guardians of their child's welfare. Thus, in most instances, the best way to protect the child's right to good mental health care is to protect the parents' rights to good information and active participation in their child's treatment. It would be overly simplistic, however, to believe that the parents' rights are *always* identical to the child's rights. There is growing awareness that in some families, the parents fail to be the best guardians of the child's welfare, and that, in such cases, the child has rights that are separate from those of the parents and that are not protected by promoting parental rights.

This chapter addresses a variety of issues that are relevant to the rights and responsibilities of parents and to the distinction between the rights of parents and the rights of children. The first section discusses parental rights to professional information and the responsibilities that flow from such rights. Following this discussion, a number of instances are described in which our society is beginning to distinguish the rights of children from the rights of their parents. A final section deals with some ways in which all parents can take responsible action to promote better mental health care for all children.

PARENTAL RIGHTS TO PROFESSIONAL INFORMATION—AND THEIR RESPONSIBILITIES CONCERNING THIS INFORMATION.

In evaluating a treatment recommendation, some parents on some occasions will feel the need to have access to professional information concerning their child. For example, parents may wish to read the psychologist's report on the psychological testing that was conducted with the child, or parents may wish to read the progress notes made by their child's therapist. Do parents have a right, legal or otherwise, to this kind of information?

Legally, there is at present no such general right. However, it must be recognized that the law in this area is rapidly changing and it is difficult to predict future legal events. As a case in point, consider some recent actions by the federal government. In the past few years, we have witnessed strong support at the federal level for the individual's right to obtain and inspect information kept on that individual by federal agencies; federal legislation has also upheld parents' rights to examine educational records kept on their children by federally supported educational institutions. Thus, there is a clear trend to facilitate people's access to their own records, but as yet this trend has not resulted in any general, nationally established parental right to inspect the records kept on their children by mental health facilities.

Regardless of the exact state of the law, however, many mental health professionals have responded to the spirit of recent legislation by personally deciding to make their records available to parents who wish to see them. Indeed, more and more mental health professionals are making a routine practice of giving copies of their reports to parents, even if no specific request for information has been made. Many professionals would therefore argue that even if this right has not been clearly *legally* established, parents do have a right to access to professional information on their child.

Rights, however, usually entail responsibilities, and such is the case in the present area. When parents are given access to professional material on their child, they must take on the responsibility of using this access wisely. Two issues seem most relevant to these responsibilities.

First of all, parents should think carefully about why they would wish to have direct access to professional information rather than having indirect access by discussing professional findings with the mental health professional. Often professional reports are written in professional jargon that will be unclear and, perhaps, confusing to a parent. Discussion, on the other hand, has the benefit of making it possible for the parent to indicate whenever anything is unclear and to obtain immediate clarification from the professional. Thus, discussion with a professional should usually give parents more information than reading a report. Probably, then, a parent would only feel the need to have direct access when the professional has not done a very good job of clarifying confusing issues, or when the parent does not trust the professional's report of what information is included in the child's file.

Another issue in having direct access to professional material concerns the child's feelings about this. Sometimes children will tell a mental health professional things that they do not want their parents to know. Parents should recognize that, in some instances, it will be possible for the professional to help the child only if the child feels free to speak openly, and some children may feel this way only if their privacy has been guaranteed by the professional. Parents who obtain direct access to professional material could then violate this privacy and could make the child feel badly, and possibly damage the relationship between the child and the professional.

Given these problems, it is a good idea for parents who believe that they may be able to obtain direct access to professional material to discuss this with their child. With younger children, violations of privacy are less likely, but once children have become old enough to value their privacy — probably somewhere around seven or eight — violations of this privacy can occur. In discussing this issue with children, parents should give them a chance to indicate, privately, to the professional any material that they do not want their parents to see; this specific material can then be withheld.

In talking about access to professional material, a final comment should be made. Professional material is confidential. Other people should not be allowed to examine this material without parental permission. In order for other people (for example, other mental health professionals at a different facility; the family's physician) to see a professional report, the parent(s) have to sign a release form authorizing this disclosure. Most mental health facilities and professionals are exceedingly careful about guarding the family's privacy, and I personally have never seen a professional report given to another person or agency without parental permission. If, however, a parent were to encounter a situation where such a report is given to another person or agency without the parent's signed permission, then the parent will want to vigorously protest this action and to consider consulting a lawyer about the possibility that the unwarranted release is grounds for bringing legal suit.[1]

THE RIGHTS OF CHILDREN

Awareness of the individual rights of children is quite recent. Traditional legal opinion holds that the parent is the guardian of the child until the child legally becomes an adult (usually age eighteen) and that no treatment (physical or psychological) can be given to the child without parental consent. Within recent years, four areas of exception to this general rule have been noted.

Child Abuse

When a child is physically or mentally abused by a parent, that parent obviously ceases to become the best guardian of the child's welfare. Within the last few years, we have begun to learn the true extent of physical abuse of children, and a number of steps have been taken to increase reporting of such abuse. Professionals who deal frequently with children have, in many states, a positive duty to report instances of physical or mental abuse of which they become aware. This professional duty and increased public

---

[1]Whether or not unwarranted release is grounds for legal action depends on whether or not the confidentiality of the professional-client relationship is protected by statute. Even where such legal guarantees do not exist, there are strong ethical constraints against unwarranted release. These constraints are upheld by all major societies of mental health professionals (for example, the American Psychological Association and the American Psychiatric Association). Thus, bringing a complaint to a professional society against a professional who reveals confidential material without permission to do so is an alternative to legal action.

concern about child abuse has led to increased reporting of such abuse, and both professionals and the general public have been shocked to learn of its frequency. It is still likely, however, that what abuse we know of is only the tip of the iceberg. In spite of their positive duty to report, many professionals are reluctant to get involved with child abuse cases. The state may grant them (and concerned nonprofessionals as well) immunity from civil prosecution (so that parents who are reported cannot sue the person who reported them), but the state cannot make up for the time and trouble that becoming involved will take (making the report, testifying, etc.), nor can the state eliminate people's concern about being wrong and reporting abuse that in fact is not occurring.

If all of these problems hamper adequate detection of physical child abuse, the situation is much worse in regard to mental abuse. It is fairly easy to get widespread agreement as to what constitutes physical abuse; it is much more difficult to get such agreement about what constitutes mental abuse. Furthermore, the signs of mental abuse are much more difficult to detect: a child who seems depressed and sad may be this way because he is emotionally abused by his parents, but it is just as probable that he is this way even though his parents have made every effort to help him be more cheerful. It is, in fact, rather seldom that any one symptom of psychological distress points directly to parental abuse or neglect. Thus while most states recognize the possibility of parents' mentally abusing their children, in practice it turns out to be only rarely that such abuse is reported to the police or the courts.

In those instances where physical (or more infrequently, mental) abuse or gross neglect is alleged, a juvenile court will investigate. If abuse or neglect is proven in court, the court can remove custody of the child from the parents. A description of juvenile courts' possible actions with regard to children's mental health is provided below.

Juvenile Courts

Children frequently come to the attention of the juvenile court through their own behavior: they may steal, be truant, get involved in a gang fight, and so forth. Whenever children come to the attention of the court, whether due to their own behavior or to reports of possible child abuse, extensive safeguards are utilized to protect the child's rights. A child appearing before a juvenile court will have, for example, his or her own attorney who is directly responsible for protecting the child's welfare and guarding the child's rights. If the court believes that a psychological disturbance may be present, it has several options:

1. It can order an evaluation of the child; it does not need parental permission to do this.
2. The court can order treatment for the child. If parents do not consent to this treatment, custody may be removed. In some cases, removal of custody will mean only that the court is in charge of the child's treatment. In other cases, the court may sever the parents' right to the child such that the parents lose completely their legal guardianship of the child.
3. If hospitalization of the child appears necessary and the parents do not consent, the court can remove custody of the child from the parents and give custody to a social services (welfare) agency, which then can hospitalize the child.
4. The court can also order treatment for the parents. If parents do not consent, custody of the child could be removed. Beyond removal of custody of the child, however, the court probably cannot enforce its order that the parents receive treatment.

It should be noted that in most instances, removal of custody is not necessary. Parents typically are most upset and worried when their child comes into contact with a juvenile court and are usually quite willing to abide by the court's orders. Removal of custody stands as an ultimate means of enforcing the court's orders, necessary for those relatively rare cases in which the parents will not follow through on the court's orders concerning the psychological treatment of their child.

Commitment Procedures

In most states, when a parent legally commits a child to an inpatient mental health facility, this commitment is treated as a voluntary admission, even though the child may not wish to enter or remain in the facility. This procedure differs considerably from that for unwilling adults. When an adult is legally committed to such a facility, this is a civil commitment. Adults who do not wish to be committed have the right to a court hearing where, represented by their own attorney, they can argue that they should not be committed. In most states at present, the unwilling child does not have such rights because regardless of the child's feelings, the commitment is legally viewed as voluntary. This state of affairs reflects the legal nonexistence of minors: if the *parents* voluntarily desire hospitalization for the child, the hospitalization is considered voluntary for the *child*. The feelings of children do not, legally, exist apart from their parents' decision.

Quite recently, a few states (such as Pennsylvania) have initiated changes in this procedure and have sought to recognize children's rights to argue against psychiatric committments desired for them by their parents. During the next few years, it is likely that this will become an important issue throughout the United States. There appears to be increasing support for providing children with the same legal protection in regard to psychiatric committment (being entitled to a court hearing and representation by their own attorney) that is now commonly extended only to adults.

Emancipated Minors

The conflict between parents' and children's rights typically becomes most acute when the child is an adolescent. In many ways, adolescents, especially older ones, are adults (certainly physically, sometimes emotionally). But legally, the adolescent before age eighteen is a child. Under some circumstances, it is possible to have a child declared an "emancipated minor." This declaration, by mutual consent of parents and child, enables the child to make certain decisions on his or her own (such as leaving a psychiatric hospital) without parental consent. Moreover, it removes parental legal obligations toward the child. If the emancipated minor runs up debts or causes damage to other people's property, the parent is not responsible. If the child were not legally an emancipated minor, the parent would be legally and thus financially responsible. Thus, while the emancipated minor procedure formally serves to enhance the child's rights, this procedure can also serve to protect parents from having to be legally and financially responsible for the child's behavior.

It should be reemphasized that this entire consideration of children's rights as separate from parental rights is a new area for the legal profession, for mental health professionals, and for society. It is a consideration that needs careful attention and examination. There is no doubt that the best guardians of children's welfare are usually their parents, but there is also no doubt that, unfortunately, there are families in which the parents do not adequately protect and promote the child's well-being. The procedures by which society better safeguards children caught in the latter situation are still evolving, and all of us, professionals and parents alike, should give such procedures our most serious consideration.

HOW TO PROMOTE QUALITY MENTAL HEALTH CARE FOR CHILDREN AND FAMILIES

Throughout this volume, I have emphasized parents' rights to have, and professionals' responsibility to provide, adequate information concerning mental health evaluation and treatment. This emphasis has reflected my belief that parents who bring their children to mental health facilities are consumers of mental health care and thus must have sufficient information to make sound decisions concerning that care. But being a consumer is a two-way street: you have the right to adequate information, but you should also assume some responsibility in working for more adequate services. Naturally this responsibility is felt most keenly by parents who have children who are receiving mental health care, but to be most effective in improving mental health care for children, *all* parents should share this responsibility. Because every parent is a *potential* consumer of mental health care for his or her child, every parent should work toward improving mental health services so that if the need ever arises, adequate care will be available.

While many, many parents would agree with the above contention, many may also be unsure about exactly what actions they can take. Mental health services are wide-ranging, offered by a number of professions in a number of different ways. What can an individual parent do to improve these services? As a partial—certainly not all-inclusive—answer to this question, I have listed some activities below that parents can engage in that can serve to increase the quality of mental health services. These activities are not listed in order of importance; nor is it suggested that every parent engage in every activity. The list is provided to give parents an idea of what sort of activities are possible, and it is hoped that individual parents will discover some activities that would interest them.

1. Join parent's groups. There are many groups formed for parents of children with specific physical and/or psychological difficulties. One does not have to be a parent of such a child to join; these groups are usually open to any interested person. These groups are also usually quite well organized and in their pursuit of better care for specific groups of children engage in a number of activities. They may, for example, work with local or state school systems, lobby government agencies, raise money for treatment and research, and provide information to parents and the general public. To find out whether a parents' group has been formed for children with a particular physical and/or psychological difficulty, parents can consult the reference librarian at any good library. The reference librarian also will be able to help parents locate the address of any national group and its regional and/or local chapter. Parents can then contact this group and find out more details about its goals and activities.

2. *Urge schools to provide mental health services.* This activity is probably especially suitable for parents who are already involved with their local school system through, for example, belonging to a PTA. Parents should find out exactly what services are offered by their local school system. One very good way to discover the answer to this question is to ask if the school system has a school psychologist and to find out how many pupils the school psychologist is responsible for. If a parent learns that there is no school psychologist, or that there is one school psychologist responsible for a very large number of children in the school district, then the parent can readily conclude that adequate services are not provided. Parents should talk with school psychologists (in their district if their district provides a school psychologist, or in any other district where a school psychologist is provided), learn what would be an adequate psychologist-pupil ratio for their district, and then work for their district's hiring a sufficient number of school psychologists. Schools have tremendous potential for the delivery of mental health care services. The children are there and, for most children, any problems they have will show up in school. Different school districts will provide different services. The principle is to get to know what is provided in *your* district and, if it does not appear to be adequate, to work to improve the services available.

3. *Work for legislation that will ensure that school districts are responsible for providing special education to those children who cannot be adequately educated in regular classrooms in regular schools.* Some states have explicitly stipulated that every child in every school district is entitled to an education. This stipulation means that districts are responsible for providing special education to those children who need it. If the district provides the special education, then the child attends school in that district. If a specific type of special education is needed by a specific child and is not provided by the district, the district is responsible for at least part of the cost of educating that child at a school that can provide the necessary type of program. Parents can check with their local superintendent of schools to see if their state has this kind of "right to education" law. If their state does not have such a law, parents can work through their local school boards and state legislators to promote legislation establishing and

protecting all children's right to an adequate education. Unless a state has recognized the right of every child to his or her needed type of education, it can be extremely difficult to establish needed special education programs. Once a state has recognized this right, getting school districts to provide needed programs is greatly facilitated.

4. Support mental health services in the community. You would have to look far and wide to find a professional who disagrees with the following statement: Providing treatment at community-based facilities is a better approach than providing treatment at facilities located at a distance from the community. Virtually all professionals think this is so, and this recognition has led to deemphasis of treatment in state hospitals and increased emphasis on treatment by community mental health centers. Community-based treatment, however, does have a problem and this problem is expense. Community services are much more expensive than a centralized institution. It will take concerted citizen action to induce states and localities to provide adequate funding for community mental health services. If parents are interested in community services, they should get in touch with their local community mental health center—or if there is not one in their community, get in touch with the nearest one. By talking with the people at these facilities, parents can find out how they can help improve community services through their role as citizens. Perhaps letters to state legislators and/or talking with a city councilman will help. Supporting bond issues that are necessary to raise money for community mental health centers will always help. If parents are interested in legal affairs, they can talk with someone who works for their local juvenile court. Juvenile courts provide substantial mental health services to the community; typically, however, they are understaffed. Working to increase the staffing and funding of the juvenile court is one way to assist in improving mental health care in the community.

5. Become aware of mental health issues in the state. If parents wish to be very active on a state level, they might visit a state psychiatric hospital and talk with the staff and patients. If they feel that the hospital provides inadequate care, they can work to improve the care through political action—talking with their state legislators, writing letters to the governor. If parents do not wish to be this active, they can at least read the newspapers carefully, look for items on mental health care, find out (either from news reports or by inquiring personally) about political candidates' views on mental health care, and then use their voting power to support those proposals or candidates that will improve mental health care in their state.

6. Support research on mental health problems. As has been noted previously in this book, our "for certain" knowledge about mental health problems is all too limited. Given this state of affairs, continued research into the causes and treatment of such problems is imperative. Research, however, requires money. Research also sometimes seems vague and incomprehensible to many people who wonder why they should spend their tax dollars on such mysterious enterprises. I think what really hinders more active citizen support of research, however, is that citizens frequently do not realize how little professionals know. I am hopeful that parents who have read this book now understand the absolute necessity for further research on human behavior and will be prepared to support this research. One can support research through giving money to charitable groups interested in children's problems, but probably the most effective support for research comes through political activity, especially at the federal level. Congressmen and senators are not accustomed to receiving letters from citizens urging support of research in mental health. Such letters can be quite influential in promoting federal support for mental health research.

URGING PROFESSIONALS
TO PROVIDE QUALITY MENTAL HEALTH CARE

While the above list of activities is quite varied and, presumably, different activities will appeal to different parents, the activity discussed in this final section is critically important for all parents who take their children to mental health professionals. Perhaps one of the best ways to introduce this activity is to return to Alice's predicament in Wonderland.

In the last chapter of *Alice's Adventures in Wonderland,* Alice rebels against the unreasonable behavior of the Queen at the trial of the Knave of Hearts.

"No, no!" said the Queen. "Sentence first—verdict afterwards."

"Stuff and nonsense!" said Alice loudly. "The idea of having the sentence first!"

"Hold your tongue!" said the Queen, turning purple.

"I won't!" said Alice.

"Off with her head!" the Queen shouted at the top of her voice. Nobody moved.
"Who cares for *you*?" said Alice (she had grown to her full size by this time). "You're nothing but a pack of cards!"

Mental health professionals are, fortunately, usually more than "a pack of cards," and they usually do not in the least resemble the inhabitants of Wonderland. Being human, however, mental health professionals are subject to the same kinds of problems that can plague any human enterprise. While most mental health professionals are well-trained and dedicated individuals, there are and always will be some exceptions. While most evaluations and treatments are carried out conscientiously and thoughtfully, there are and always will be some that are not. Parents who have read this book should now be able to recognize inadequate, superficial, or careless mental health care should they be so unfortunate as to encounter it. In such cases, "Stuff and nonsense!" is not a bad phrase to have available. Parents should demand quality mental health care for themselves and for their children. If the services they receive are poor in quality, parents should make it clear that they will not purchase such services and will go elsewhere if necessary. People tend to live up to the expectations that others have of them. When parents expect and insist on the best mental health care, mental health professionals will tend to "try harder" to provide it.

Index

Ability tests, 65-66
Abramowitz, C. V., 101
Adolescence, mental health problems in, 26-36
Aggression, 16, 24-25, 31, 37
Alcohol, 32-35
Ames, L., 10
Amphetamines, 33-35
Anorexia nervosa, 29-30
Aphasia, developmental, 19-20
Articulation problems, 18
Assessment of mental health problems, 59-74
Autism, 13-14

Barbiturates, 33-35
Behavior problems:
 during adolescence, 29-30
 during elementary school years, 23-25
 during preschool years, 15-17
 example of evaluation of 73-74
Behavior therapy, 82-85
 desensitization, 84-85
 evaluation of recommendation for, 110

Behavior therapy (continued):
 reinforcement management, 83
 time-out, 83
Bender, L., 128
Benefit-harm ratio, 103, 109-110, 112-113, 114-115, 119
Bergin, A.E., 99
Brain, traumatic injury to, 35

Child abuse, 157-158
Child guidance clinics, 45-46
Child-rearing counseling, 85, 110
Client-centered therapy, 80-81
Cocaine, 33-35
Commitment procedures, 159
Communication disorders:
 during adolescence, 35-36
 during elementary school years, 25
 during preschool years, 18-20
Community mental health centers, 46-47
Community mental health services, 163

168 Index

Consulting mental health professionals
  emotional barriers, 39-41
  practical difficulties, 41
  second opinions, 94-95
Consumers:
  of mental health services, 4-5
  of other services and products, 4
Corey, G., 78
Couples therapy (see Psychotherapy)
Crisis centers, 41-42

Depression, 28-29, 37-38
Desensitization (see Behavior therapy)
Developmental evaluation clinics, 43
Discussions about mental health services
  with child, 132-141
  with other family members, 142-143
Down's syndrome, 12
Drug-related problems, 32-35

Eating problems, 16, 24, 29-30
Educational consultants, 57
Electro-convulsive therapy (ECT), 90, 122-123
  evaluating a treatment recommendation
  for, 127-129
Elementary school years, mental health
  problems in, 20-26
Elimination, problems with, 24
Emancipated minors, 160
Emergency situations, 41-42
Emotional disturbance, 140
  during adolescence, 29
  during elementary school years, 22-23
  during preschool years, 15
Enuresis, 24, 140
Erickson, M., 10
Evaluation:
  of child's problem by mental health
    professionals, 59-74
  of treatment effectiveness by mental health
    professionals, 103-105, 109-110, 113,
    115, 120
  of treatment recommendation by parents,
    92-131

Family therapy (see Psychotherapy)
Freud, A., 79
Freud, S., 3, 52n, 78, 92
  (see also Psychoanalysis)

Glue-sniffing, 33-35
Group homes, 48
Group therapy (see Psychotherapy)

Heroin, 33-35
Horney, K., 79
Hot-lines (see Crisis centers)
Hydrocephaly, 12
Hyperactivity, 17, 25, 115-119

Ilg, F., 10
Individual therapy (see Psychotherapy)
Inpatient treatment, 88-90
  evaluating treatment recommendation
    for, 119-130
  permanent residence, 123-130
  short-term, 120-123
  physical treatments, 88-90, 127-130
  psychological treatments, 89, 126-127
Institutionalization, 123-130
Intellectual development (see Mental
  retardation)
Intelligence testing, 60-65
Interpersonal therapy, 79
Interviews, 59-60
Inventories, 67-68
IQ (see Intelligence testing)

Jung, C., 3
Juvenile courts, 158-159, 163

Klein, M., 79

Learning disability, 139-140
  during adolescence, 27
  during elementary school years, 21-22
  example of evaluation of, 71-73
Levitt, E.E., 100
LSD, 32-35

Manic-depression, 28-29
  (see also Depression)
Marijuana, 32-35
Medical model, 3
Medication, 17, 87-90, 127
  evaluating treatment recommendation
    for, 113-119

Index 169

Mental health problems of children:
  characteristics of, 8-9
  types of, 10-36
Mental retardation, 139
  during adolescence, 26-27
  during elementary school years, 21-22
  during preschool years, 11-13
  example of evaluation of, 70-71
Modification of parental expectations, 76, 96-99
Mongolism (see Down's syndrome)

Neurologists, 56
Normal development, 9-10
Note-taking on child's behavior, 36-38
Nurses:
  LPN's, 55
  RN's, 54-55

Obesity (see Eating problems)
Observation, 68-69
Occupational therapists, 57

Parent Effectiveness Training (PET), 85, 110
Parents' groups, 45, 161-162
Patterson, G. R., 84
Paying for mental health services, 144-153
  evaluations:
    inpatient, 148-149
    outpatient, 144-146
  governmental assistance programs, 145-146
  insurance, 145-151
  sliding scale fee system, 145-149
  treatment:
    inpatient, 149-151
    outpatient, 146-148
Pediatricians, 42
  for assistance with elementary school age problems, 20-36
  for assistance with preschool problems, 11-20
  training and description of skills, 56
Phenylketonuria, 12
Physical therapists, 57
Physically handicapped children, mental health problems of
  during adolescence, 36
  during elementary school years, 26
  during preschool years, 20

PKU (see Phenylketonuria)
Play therapy (see Psychotherapy)
Preschool years, mental health problems in, 10-20
Private practitioners, 44-45
Private psychiatric hospitals, 49, 150
Professional information, parents' rights to, 4, 155-157
Projective tests, 66-67
Psychiatric aides or attendants, 55
Psychiatrists, 44-45, 51-52
Psychiatry, departments of, 47
Psychoanalysis, 52n, 78-79, 80
Psychoanalysts, 52
Psychologists, 44-45, 52-53
Psychosis:
  during adolescence, 27-29
  during elementary school years, 22
  during preschool years, 13-15
Psychosurgery, 90, 122-123
  evaluating a treatment recommendation for, 129-130
Psychotherapy:
  effectiveness, 99-100
  evaluating a treatment recommendation for, 102-105
  forms of:
    couples therapy, 81
    family therapy, 82, 101-102
    group therapy, 82, 101
    individual therapy, 80-81, 100-101
    play therapy, 81
  theories of, 78-80

Rehabilitation, 56
Reinforcement management (see Behavior therapy)
Research on mental health problems, 92-93, 164
Ritalin, 87-88
Rogers, C., 4, 80
Ross, D., 113
Ross, S., 113

Schizophrenia:
  during adolescence, 27-28
  during childhood, 14-15
School phobia, 23
School psychologists, 21-22, 162
  (see also Psychologists, Special education)
Schools, mental health services in, 162-163
  (see also Special education)

Schools for emotionally disturbed children, 49
Second opinions, 94-95
Sexual problems, 31-32
Sleep disturbances, 16, 24, 30
Social workers, 44-45, 53-54
Special education, 85-87
  evaluating a treatment recommendation for, 111-113
Speech:
  delay, 19
  development, 12-13
  problems (see Communication disorders)
Speech and language specialists, 56-57
  (see also Communication disorders, Speech)
State hospitals, 48-49, 149-150
State mental health services, 163-164
Stuttering, 18, 35
Suicide, 41
  (see also Depression)
Sullivan, H.S., 3, 79
Supplementary:
  evaluations, 69-70
  treatments, 90-91, 130-131
Supportive therapy, 85, 110-111

Team approach, 57-58
Tests (see Ability tests, Intelligence testing, Inventories, Projective tests)
Time-out (see Behavior therapy)
Timidity, 17, 25, 31
Toilet-training, 16
Treatment of mental health problems:
  evaluating recommendations for, 92-131
  types of, 75-92

Urging professionals to provide quality mental health care, 164-165

Veterans Administration hospitals, 47-48

Wolpe, J., 106